live Better ashtanga yoga

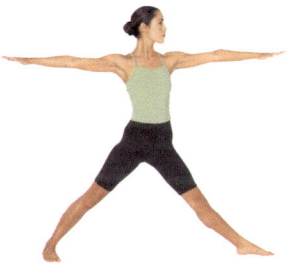

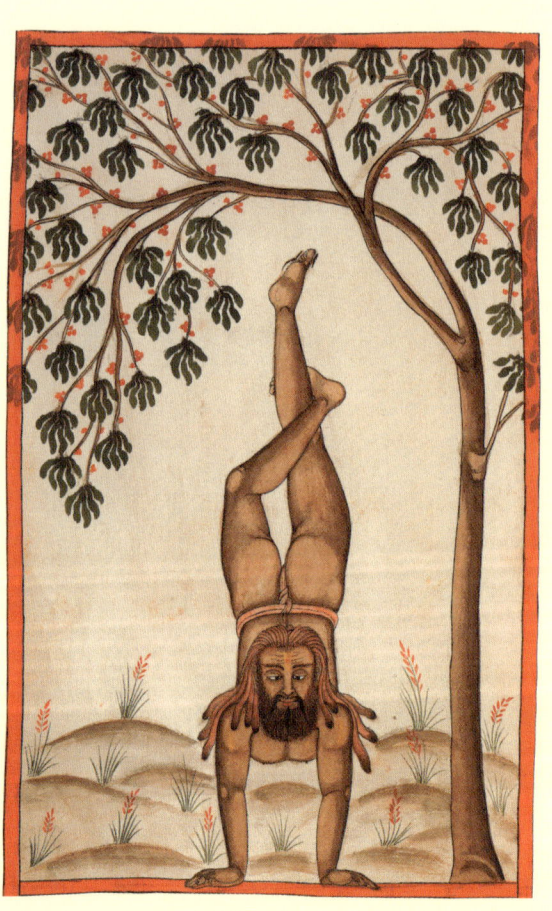

live Better ashtanga yoga

exercises and inspirations for well-being

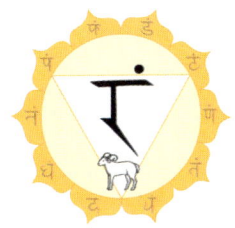

Anton Simmha

DUNCAN BAIRD PUBLISHERS

LONDON

Live Better: Ashtanga Yoga
Anton Simmha

With love and respect to the memory of
Derek Ireland and the global Ashtanga family.

First published in Canada in 2003 by
Raincoast Books
9050 Shaughnessy Street
Vancouver, B.C.
V6P 6E5
(604) 323-7100
www.raincoast.com

Conceived, created, and designed by
Duncan Baird Publishers Ltd.
Sixth Floor, Castle House
75–76 Wells Street
London W1T 3QH

Managing Editor: Judy Barratt
Editor: Lucy Latchmore
Managing Designer: Manisha Patel
Designer: Allan Sommerville
Picture Research: Cecilia Weston-Baker
Commissioned Photography: Matthew Ward

Cataloging-in-publication data available
from the publisher

10 9 8 7 6 5 4 3 2 1

ISBN: 1-904292-31-3

Typeset in Filosofia and Son Kern
Color reproduction by Scanhouse, Malaysia
Printed and bound by Imago, Thailand

PUBLISHER'S NOTE
Before following any advice or practice
suggested in this book, it is recommended that
you consult your doctor as to its suitability,
especially if you suffer from any health
problems or special conditions. The
publishers, the author, and the photographers
cannot accept any responsibility for any
injuries or damage incurred as a result of
following the exercises in this book, or of
using any of the therapeutic techniques
described or mentioned here.

contents

INTRODUCTION

My path toward Ashtanga yoga began during the late 1980s, while I was working in London as an artist and designer. At the time my main preoccupation was partying – something that I did with a passion bordering on the extreme. But after years of extreme living, I had pushed my body to the limits of physical endurance and abuse. I knew that I had to change my lifestyle radically, and so I began a search for balance and peace that was to be the beginning of my spiritual awakening.

At this point I had been practising yoga in London, on and off, for a couple of years. Then, while on holiday in Goa, South India, I was fortunate enough to meet an extraordinary man, called Derek Ireland, who introduced me to a form of yoga that I had never seen before – Ashtanga *Vinyasa* yoga!

Inspired by watching Derek perform this graceful practice on the beach, the "yoga penny" finally dropped. I suddenly knew that Ashtanga was the answer if I wanted to heal my body, my mind and my spirit.

The purpose of this book is to introduce you to the practice and concepts of Ashtanga *Vinyasa* yoga, in the hope that yoga may help you as it has helped me. It is intended as a beginner's introduction to the discipline and contains an abbreviated version of the Primary Series – the foundation sequence of Ashtanga yoga.

It is important to stress that this book should serve only as an aid to your practice, giving you some introductory insights into the purpose, techniques and benefits of this ancient system. It should not be used as a replacement for a qualified teacher.

Before attempting any of the exercises in this book, read the text all the way through to gain an overview of the subject. When you come to the exercises, read them through twice. The second time visualize yourself doing each step in turn to help you remember them better.

Above all, always follow this fundamental rule: never force, never stress, never strain, never overexert. Learn to listen to your body – it will always tell you how far to go.

Good luck. *Namaste* – Anton

about ashtanga

Ashtanga *Vinyasa* yoga is a form of Hatha (physical) yoga that, like other physical forms, uses postures and breathing techniques as a starting point for attaining a state of "yoga" or "union". This is the ultimate goal of any type of yoga and involves the yoking together of mind, body and spirit so that we can experience self-realization or enlightenment.

Ashtanga yoga is unique in its use of *vinyasas* (breath-synchronized movements), which link the yoga postures together to form dynamic sequences. This book covers four sequences of postures, which together comprise a basic form of the Primary Series. This is the first of six Ashtanga series, the others being the Intermediate Series and Advanced Series A, B, C and D. The Primary Series is sometimes called "Yoga Chikitsa", meaning "Yoga Therapy". This name refers to the healing nature of the series, which aims to create a strong, light, energetic body and a clear and focused mind in preparation for the more demanding postures of later series.

In this chapter we trace the history, aims and philosophy of Ashtanga yoga, the specific techniques that this form involves and the range of benefits these can bring you — whether you want to improve your fitness and flexibility or, on a deeper level, seek more spiritual meaning in your life.

A BRIEF HISTORY OF ASHTANGA

Yoga is a living tradition, which emerged during the ancient Vedic civilization of India around 2800BCE. Throughout the centuries this tradition has been preserved by generations of teachers, who have passed on their wisdom verbally to their students. A number of these teachers have developed their own individual styles of yoga, resulting in the various different forms of the practice in existence today.

Ashtanga *Vinyasa* yoga is based on the teachings of a celebrated guru called Sri T Krishnamacharya and was popularized in the latter part of the twentieth century by its principal proponent and modern-day guru, Sri K Pattabhi Jois of Mysore, South India.

Pattabhi Jois (or Guruji as he is known by his students) began studying yoga under the tutelage of Sri T Krishnamacharya at the age of twelve in 1927. It is reputed that during the 1930s Krishnamacharya was carrying out research in the university library of Calcutta when he discovered an ancient Sanskrit manuscript called the *Yoga Korunta*, written by an ancient seer called Vamana Rishi. The exact age of this document remains shrouded in mystery, but it is believed to be somewhere between two thousand and five thousand years old.

With the help of Guruji (also a Sanskrit scholar), Krishnamacharya translated the *Yoga Korunta* to reveal the outline of Ashtanga *Vinyasa* yoga – a form of yoga based on a detailed system of counting breaths into and out of postures, combined with ordered sequences of movement. Guruji has become the principal teacher of this form of yoga, and is the founder of the Ashtanga Yoga Research Institute, which conducts research into the health benefits of Ashtanga.

During the 1960s and 1970s, increasing numbers of Westerners travelled to India in search of alternative ways of life. A few of these individuals trained with Guruji in Mysore and were later responsible for introducing Ashtanga to the West. Since then this dynamic and physically challenging type of yoga has become popular in many countries around the world, as people look for holistic approaches to health and fitness.

THE EIGHT LIMBS OF ASHTANGA

The word "Ashtanga" derives from the Sanskrit *ast*, meaning "eight", and *anga*, meaning "limbs". It refers to the systematic approach to life outlined in the *Yoga Sutras* – an important yogic text written by the sage Patanjali, between 200BCE and 200CE.

Patanjali envisioned the eight limbs of yoga as the interconnecting branches of a tree. *Asana* (posture practice) and *pranayama* (controlled breathing) are two of these limbs. The remaining six limbs are *yama* (ethics), *niyama* (self-discipline), *pratyahara* (withdrawal of the senses), *dharana* (concentration), *dhyana* (meditation) and *samadhi* (union with the true self). Working on any one limb encourages the others to grow in turn, leading ultimately toward enlightenment.

Ashtanga yoga focuses initially on *asana* and *pranayama* (covered in chapters two to five). As your practice develops you may wish to draw on the remaining six limbs (discussed in chapter six) in order to extend yoga into other areas of your life.

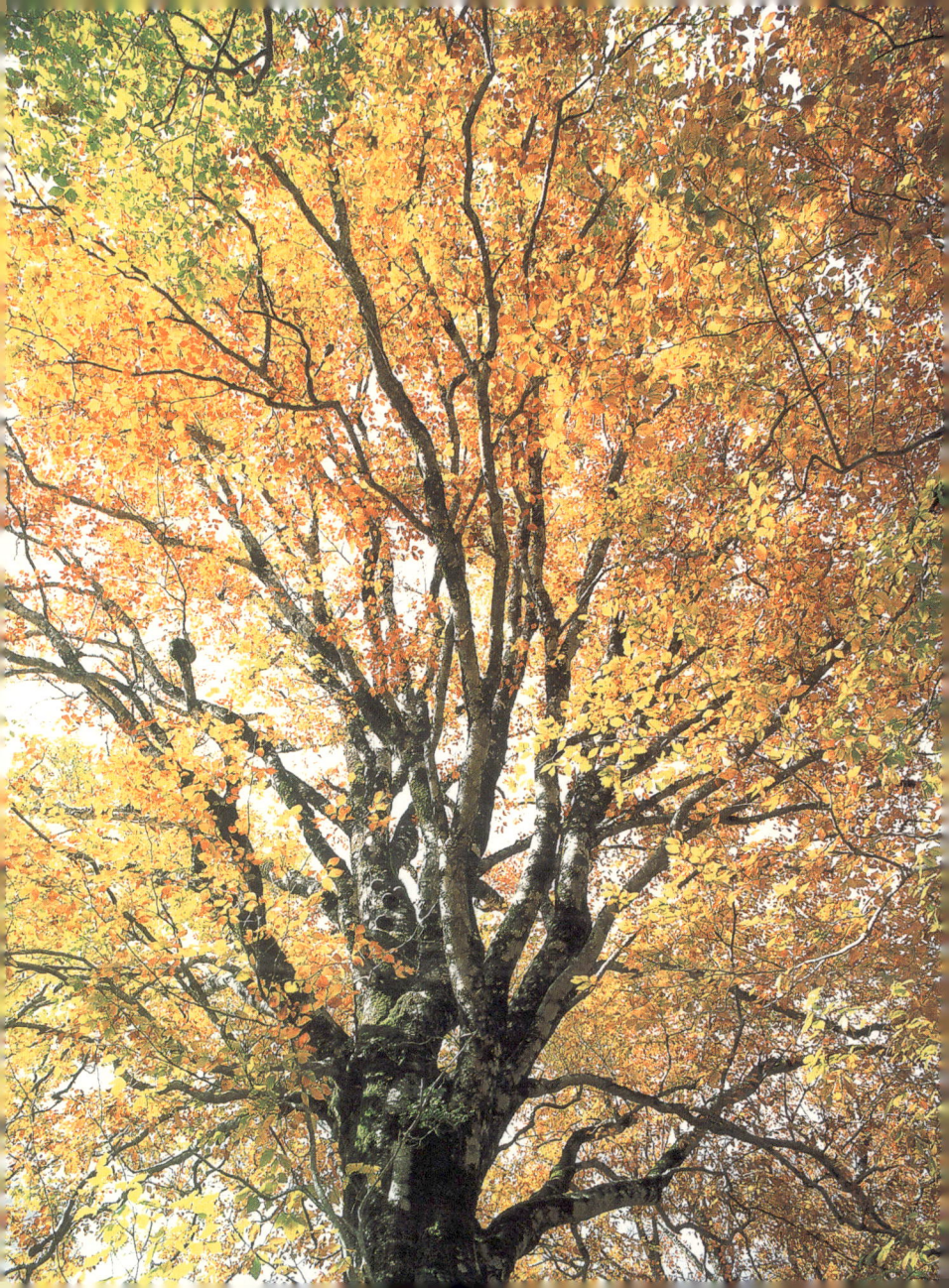

SEEKING BALANCE

As children we exist "freely" – in a natural state of balance between mind and body in which thought and movement are seamless. As we grow into adulthood, most of us are conditioned to focus on the mind's capabilities at the expense of the body's and our natural state of balance is lost.

As we move and breathe in the practice of yoga, we reestablish the balance between mind and body. The ancient yogis explained this realignment with reference to what they called the three "Bodies of Man": the Physical Body (called Stula), the Astral or Subtle Body (Sukshma) and the Causal Body (Karana). Each of these bodies comprises one or more "sheaths", of which there are five in total. The Physical Body has only one sheath, the food sheath (known as the *annamaya kosha*). The Astral Body comprises three sheaths: the pranic or vital sheath (*pranamaya kosha*), the mental sheath (*manomaya kosha*) and the intellectual sheath (*vijnana-maya kosha*). The Causal Body has one sheath, called the blissful sheath (*anandamaya kosha*). The five sheaths fit together like the layers of a Russian doll, one inside the other, with the *annamaya kosha* the outermost and the *anandamaya kosha* the innermost.

Through the practice of Ashtanga yoga, we aim to bring into balance each of the bodies and their respective sheaths in order to reconnect with the *bindu*, the seed of the true self that lies at the centre of the *anandamaya kosha*. We do this initially by combining the controlled rhythm of *pranayama* breathing with the *vinyasa* movements of Ashtanga to encourage the body to relax, stretch and open. This helps us to move safely into the physical postures of yoga, which realign and strengthen our skeletal and muscular structures, stimulate and cleanse our internal organs and enhance the flow of energy throughout the body as a whole.

By focusing our attention entirely on the rhythm of the breath and the synchronized movements of the body, we learn to still the mind, centring it within the body. In so doing, the mind and the body become one as we move toward the state of "yoga" or "union".

THE BODY'S ENERGY SYSTEM

Ancient yogis described the structure of the vital sheath (*pranamaya kosha*) as a network of interconnecting energy channels called the "subtle anatomy" – a system similar to the meridian networks of Chinese medicine. In the yogic tradition these channels are called *nadis* and distribute *prana* (vital life force) throughout the body.

It is believed that there are 72,000 *nadis*. The most important is the *sushumna nadi*, a central pranic tube that runs the length of the spinal column, from the perineum, below the groin, up to the crown of the head. Two other major *nadis* – the *ida* and *pingala* – crisscross the *sushumna nadi* and connect to the left and right nostrils respectively. These channels intersect with the *sushumna nadi* at seven key points called *chakras*. The *chakras* are the main energy centres of the body and their positions correspond to the various nerve plexuses of the spinal cord (see illustration, p.19). The *chakras* distribute energy throughout the subtle anatomy and can be envisaged as spinning spheres of light.

The breathing techniques and postures of yoga help to balance the flow of *prana* through the vital sheath. When we inhale in a controlled fashion through our nostrils, *prana* enters the *ida* and *pingala nadis*, where it is distributed throughout the energetic system. Performing the postures stimulates the movement of the *prana* through the *nadis* and *chakras*, clearing the blockages that often result from the stresses of Western living.

The Chakras

- The red *muladhara* or root *chakra* is located by the perineum, at the base of the spine. It symbolizes our primal connection to the earth element. Focusing upon it grounds us, giving a sense of security and belonging.
- The orange *swadhisthana* or sacral *chakra* is located just above the genitals and symbolizes our place of origin. Its energy governs sexuality and creativity, and it corresponds to the water element.
- The yellow *manipura* or solar plexus *chakra* lies behind the navel, at our centre. It connects us with the energy of the sun and provides us with the impetus for all our

actions – it is the source of our willpower. It also correlates to the fire element: by focusing on the *manipura chakra* we can stoke our *agni* or "internal fire".

- The green *anahata* (heart) *chakra* is situated close to the heart organ in the central chest area. This is the emotional centre of the body – the seat of compassion and unconditional love – and relates to the air element.

- The blue throat *chakra* is called *vishuddha*, meaning purity. Located at the base of the neck, it is the centre of expression and knowledge and is governed by ether.

- The purple "third eye" *chakra* is called *ajna*, meaning "inner eye", and is located in the middle of the fore-head, just above the eyebrows. It is the centre for spiritual vision, ruling our intellectual thought processes and connecting us to the wisdom of the cosmos.

- The crown *chakra* on top of the head is called *sahasrara*, which means "a thousand petals". It is depicted as a full-blossomed lotus flower and is believed to radiate a thousand rays of light from its centre. This *chakra* connects us to the universal consciousness, and meditating on it moves us toward a realization of our true selves.

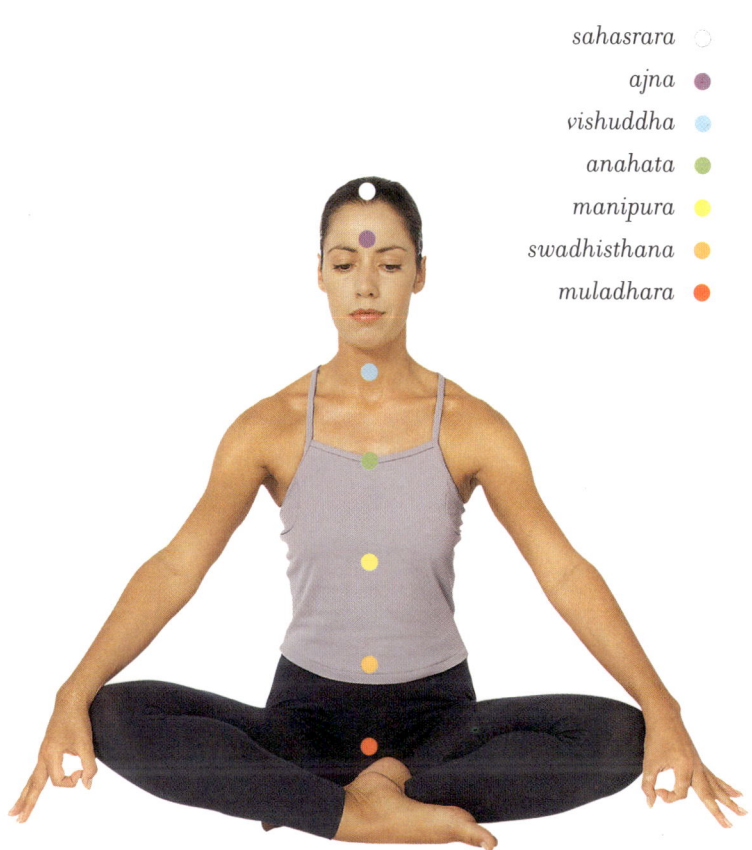

sahasrara
ajna
vishuddha
anahata
manipura
swadhisthana
muladhara

THE VINYASA SYSTEM

It is the *vinyasa* system that makes Ashtanga *Vinyasa* yoga unique. The term *vinyasa* refers to the breath-synchronized movements that link the various yoga postures together, creating a "dynamic flow" throughout the practice. This fluidity of movement and breathing differentiates Ashtanga from other forms of Hatha yoga, in which rests are often taken between postures.

One of the main functions of the *vinyasa* system is to generate an intense heat called *agni* within the internal organs that will then permeate throughout the rest of the body. The benefits of this heat are twofold: first, it is deeply purifying, encouraging the body to release toxins as sweat through the skin; second, it encourages the body to become more malleable, like heated metal, enabling it to stretch with minimum risk of injury.

The Vinyasa Movement

The *vinyasa* movement is in fact a sequence of movements. The *vinyasa* itself is based on sun salutation A (see pp.38–41), a sequence of movements that is often performed several times at the start of a yoga session. In addition to heating the body, practising these movements helps us to develop strength and stamina throughout the upper torso as well as realigning the skeletal and muscular structures of the body after each posture. Beginners can find the *vinyasa* movement rather challenging at first, so I have omitted the *vinyasas* between the standing postures (with the exception of the warrior sequence; see pp.66-71) and have included a modified version of the half-*vinyasa* (see pp.76–7), to be practised after each sitting posture (or after each side of each sitting posture when you feel ready).

The Vinyasa Breath

The breathing technique used synchronistically within both the *vinyasa* movements and the postures that they link is called *ujjayi*, which means "victorious". The aim is to sustain this form of breathing throughout the course of the yoga practice, synchronizing every movement with either an inhalation or an exhalation. In each case the impulse to move originates with the breath. The exercises in chapters two to five explain how the various movements fit together with the breathing.

When we practise *ujjayi* breathing, we create a unique sound in the back of the throat that is reminiscent of the rush of distant waves. We can create this sound by breathing through the nostrils, softening the palate and narrowing the epiglottis (the aperture at the back of the throat). This narrowing catches the breath momentarily, enabling us to control the breath as it flows into and out of our lungs. We are aiming to keep each in-breath and out-breath identical in terms of both duration and effort. When this is achieved the breathing cycle becomes more circular as the natural pauses between breaths diminish, creating a rolling breath that leaves no real distinction between inhalations and exhalations.

To experience your own *ujjayi* sound, sit in a comfortable and relaxed position, place your hands over your ears and breathe in and out, sighing audibly with your mouth open. This will produce an "ahh" and a "haa" sound. Once you can do this successfully, close your mouth and breathe through your nose, but continue to make the "ahh" and "haa" sounds by maintaining the slight constriction at the back of your throat. Breathe within your normal capacity – you are trying to create an even and relaxed breath, so do not puff up your chest or force the exhalation. Allow your entire ribcage to open as you breathe into the front, sides and back of your upper chest, expanding your lungs fully. As you do so try to keep your abdomen soft and still, lightly drawn in and up without locking it tight. This will create a bridge of support for your internal organs during your practice.

When you first begin practising Ashtanga yoga, you will probably find that most of your attention is occupied with following the sequence of movements for each exercise. However, when these become more familiar you will be able to direct more of your attention to synchronizing your movements with the breath. Try to focus on the rushing sound of the *ujjayi* breath, treating it like a mantra. This will transform your practice into a moving meditation that quietens your thoughts and emotions, enhancing your internal awareness.

THE BANDHAS

As you become more familiar with the movements and breathing of the *vinyasa* system, try to incorporate the *bandhas* into your yoga practice. *Bandha* is a Sanskrit word meaning "to lock, catch or seal". In terms of Ashtanga yoga, the *bandhas* are internal locks created by the gentle contraction of muscles within specific areas of the body. These function rather like valves, working together to contain and direct *prana* upward through the *nadis* of the subtle anatomy. Holding these locks provides the extra energy necessary for sustaining the momentum of an Ashtanga practice and helps to contain the heat generated by the *vinyasas*. In physical terms *bandhas* support the lower back and internal organs as well as aiding *ujjayi* breathing.

There are three *bandhas* used in Ashtanga: *mula bandha* or root lock, *uddiyana bandha* or lower abdominal lock and *jalandhara bandha*, throat lock. *Mula bandha* is achieved at the base of the spine and is responsible for retaining *prana* within the body. You can locate it by drawing up the muscles of the anal sphincter at the end of an exhalation. As you become more sensitive in this area, you will find that your awareness shifts slightly forward to your perineum, just below the genitals.

Uddiyana bandha is achieved in the lower abdominal region. When held it encourages *prana* to flow upward through the *nadis* of the subtle anatomy. To locate this lock draw your abdomen in and up at the end of an exhalation, when your lungs are empty. Continue to hold your abdomen in this position as you inhale – you are aiming for a soft stillness (not a hard crunching) in your lower belly that you can sustain during your practice.

Jalandhara bandha is a throat lock that is engaged when practising certain *pranayama* techniques. You should practise it only under qualified supervision.

Initially it is difficult to grasp the subtlety of the *bandhas* without the help of a teacher, but with practice you will find them easier to locate and sustain during your yoga sessions. When you do you will find that they transform your practice, giving you an internal strength and lightness that enhances every movement.

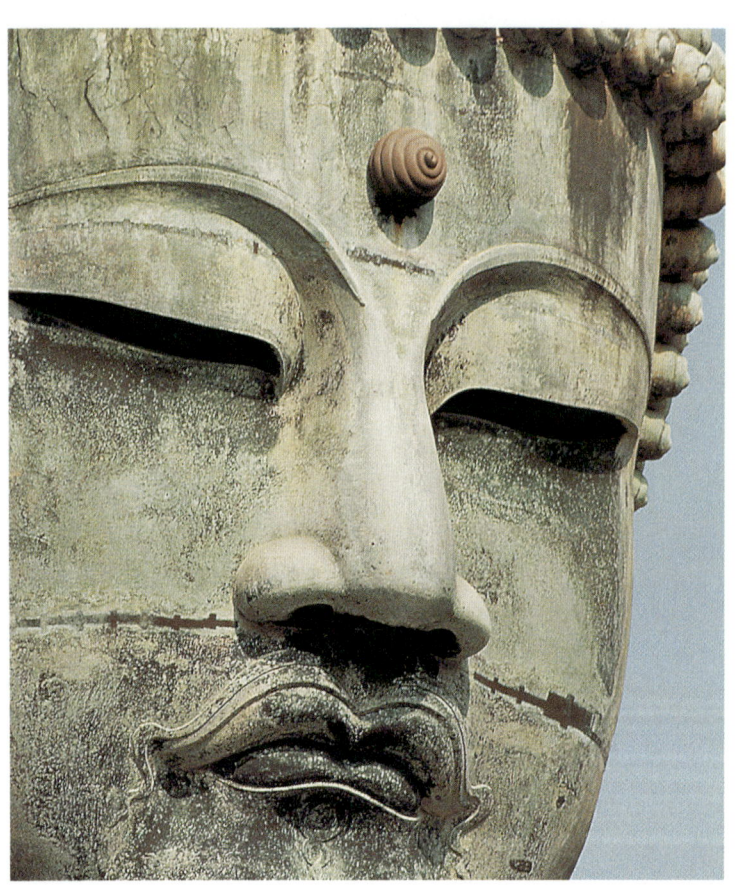

THE DRISHTIS

In each of the exercises in the book, you will find that as
you hold each posture you are instructed to look toward
certain points on your body or in your surroundings.
These gaze points are called *drishtis*. Focusing on these
points during your practice will prevent your eyes from
wandering around your surroundings. This helps the
mind to concentrate and to develop a deeper internal
focus on the body – on the action of the *ujjayi* breath,
the physical movements of the postures, the muscular
contractions of the *bandhas* and any other sensations
that arise during your practice.

Ashtanga yoga uses nine *drishtis*, which you will find
referred to in each of the exercises. These are as follows:
the tip of the nose (*nasagrai*); the thumbs (*angusta
ma dyai*); the "third eye" (*broomadhya*), located in the
middle of the forehead, just above the eyebrows;
the navel (*nabi*); up to the sky (*urdhva*); the hand
(*hastagrai*); the toes (*padhayoragrai*); the far left (*parsva*);
and the far right (*parsva*).

ATTITUDES TO YOUR PRACTICE

If yoga is to benefit you, it is important to cultivate healthy attitudes toward your practice. Ashtanga is a physically challenging form of yoga, so it is important to develop sensitivity toward your body. Such awareness will ensure the safety of your practice, helping you to find and maintain correct postural alignment and to avoid overstraining your muscles.

Before embarking upon a yoga session, take a few moments to tune into your body, checking for any areas of pain or tension. Where these exist you may need to adapt your practice accordingly, avoiding any postures that could aggravate your condition. While one of the reasons for practising yoga is to challenge ourselves, we should do so without causing pain or injury. To do this we must be aware of our limits within each posture. When easing yourself into a posture, you will discover what are known as your "minimum edge" and "maximum edge". Your minimum edge is the point at which you first feel a stretch in a posture. Your maximum edge is your "surrender point" – the furthest you can stretch before you come up against your body's natural wall of resistance. If you force your body to stretch beyond this point, you may experience pain or discomfort and risk injuring yourself. Instead try to relax into the position by focusing on your breathing. This is called "dying to the pose" or "surrendering to the breath", and it allows your body to expand its natural limits at its own pace, without causing any damage.

By letting the wisdom of your body take charge of your practice, you move beyond the desires and expect-ations of your ego, which seeks to push your body beyond its limits for the sake of immediate achievement. It is more beneficial to focus on the state of your body in the present, allowing it to relax and open of its own accord.

This attitude of patience is also essential when deal-ing with the mind. During your practice you may notice your attention wandering. Try not to become frustrated with yourself. Instead simply return your focus to your breathing. This will quieten the mind's activity, return-ing you to the present moment in your body.

KEY POINTS FOR PRACTICE

1   Wait at least two hours after a heavy meal before practising yoga, and in the first hour after your session eat
only lightly. During your practice keep drinking to a
minimum, taking only a few sips of water if you need to.

2   If possible allocate a set time each day in which to
practise yoga. The ideal time is first thing in the morning, but if this is not possible simply choose the time
that is most convenient for you.

3   Try to practise regularly. Remember that little and often
is better than sessions that are longer but infrequent.

4   Practise yoga in a well-heated room. This will ensure
that you maintain enough internal body heat to prevent
your muscles from becoming cold, thereby reducing the
risk of injury.

5   Create a soothing environment to help you to relax. Try
lighting some candles or burning some incense.

6   Try to minimize distractions during your yoga session.
Choose a quiet room in which to practise and switch off
your television, radio, telephone and mobile phone.

7 Wear light, loose, comfortable clothing and remove your shoes and socks, your watch and any jewelry.

8 Buy a yoga mat. This will provide you with a safe, nonslip surface on which to work.

9 When trying Ashtanga yoga for the first time, build up your practice slowly. Begin by doing the sun salutations from the Warm-up Sequence, followed by the cool-down poses from the Finishing Sequence. Gradually incorporate the standing postures and the floor postures as you feel your strength and stamina increasing.

10 Use your breath as a guide. If your breathing has quickened, you are probably trying too hard. Pause and relax for a moment. Reestablish an even rhythm in your breathing before continuing with your practice.

11 If you feel faint or light-headed, stop and rest.

12 Look for a yoga class or teacher in your area. This will be invaluable for developing your practice further.

13 If you are pregnant, feel unwell or have a medical condition, seek the advice of your doctor before beginning an unsupervised yoga practice.

14 Have fun!

... Our yesterdays are but dreams
Our tomorrows merely visions
But today lived well makes
Every yesterday a dream of joy,
And each tomorrow a vision of promise ...

ATTRIBUTED TO KALIDASA

SANSKRIT POEM "THE SALUTATION OF THE DAWN" (5TH CENTURY CE)

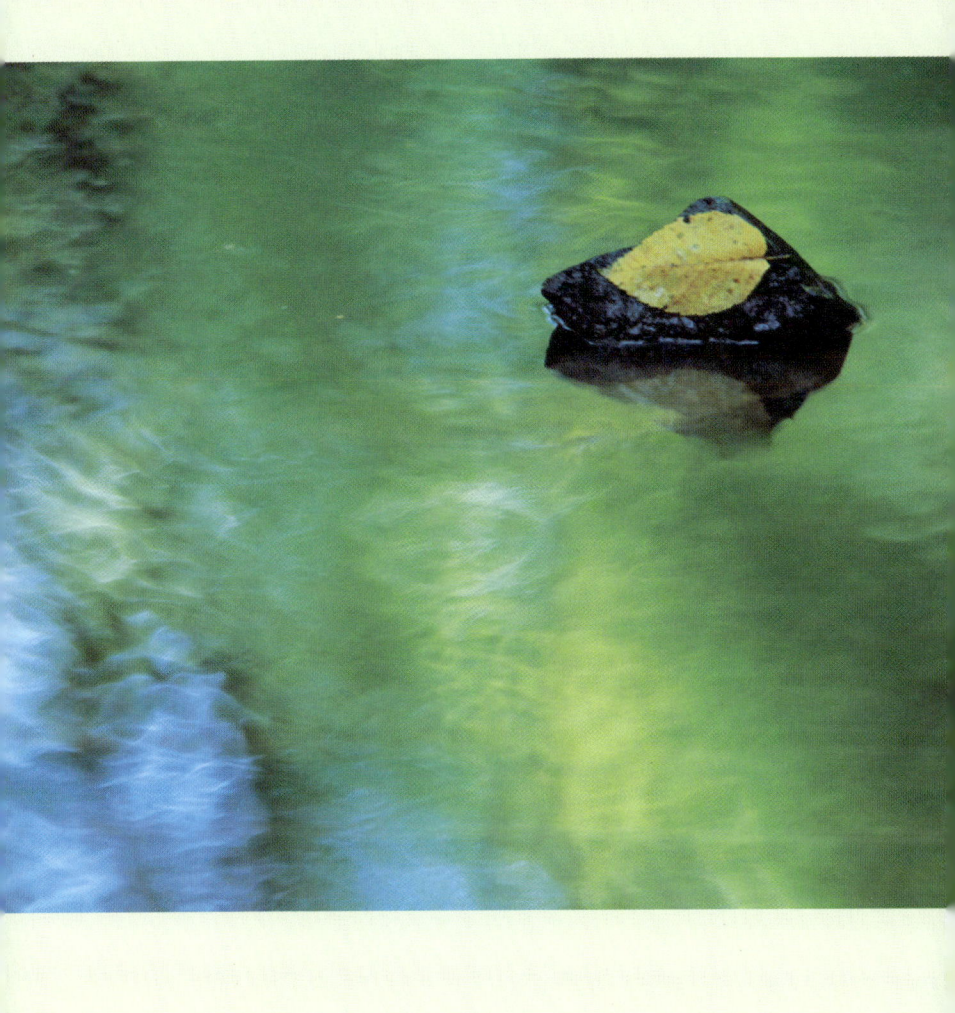

the warm-up sequence

The Warm-up Sequence is composed of two sets of movements called sun salutation A and sun salutation B. These are repeated several times at the beginning of a practice and in modifed forms later on. The sun salutations comprise a series of movements synchronized with *ujjayi* breathing and, as such, form the basis for the *vinyasa* (see pp.20–23). Performed at the beginning of an Ashtanga practice, they serve to generate *agni*, or internal heat, within our bodies. This heat increases our flexibility, allowing us to open up our bodies safely and effectively during the posture sequences without straining muscles or damaging ligaments and tendons.

The Warm-up Sequence is the foundation stone of the Ashtanga practice. It is also the perfect training ground for beginners, teaching us how to connect up the breath and the movements of the *vinyasa* system. The first few times that you practise the Warm-up Sequence, concentrate on mastering sun salutation A, before attempting the more complex sun salutation B. To begin with, repeat the sun salutations three times each, increasing the number of repetitions to five as your fitness, strength and flexibility improves.

Try practising sun salutations in the mornings before breakfast – they will increase your energy levels and concentration for the rest of the day.

The Lord of Love lies beyond and yet within us.
He is unborn, without body and mind, name or form.
Yet he is the source of all:
Space, air, fire, water and earth –
The elements from which life is created.

MUNDAKA UPANISHAD (5TH CENTURY BCE)

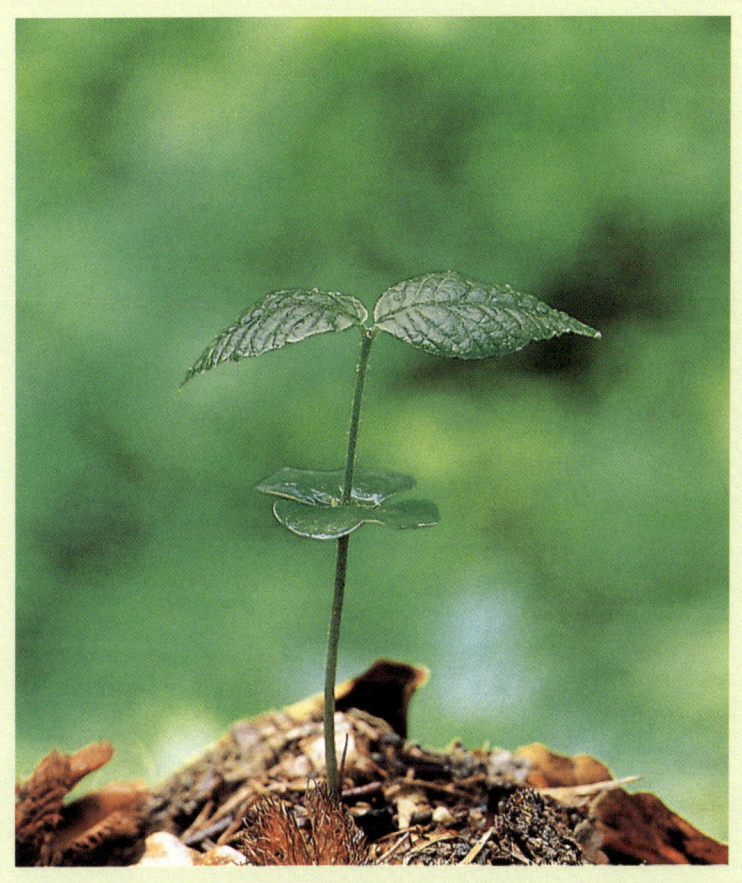

SUN SALUTATION A
Surya Namaskara A

Adopt standing ready pose (*samasthiti*) with your feet together, arms by your sides and shoulders relaxed. Begin even and relaxed *ujjayi* breathing.

1   Inhaling, take your arms out to the side and bring them up above your head with your palms together. Look up at your thumbs.

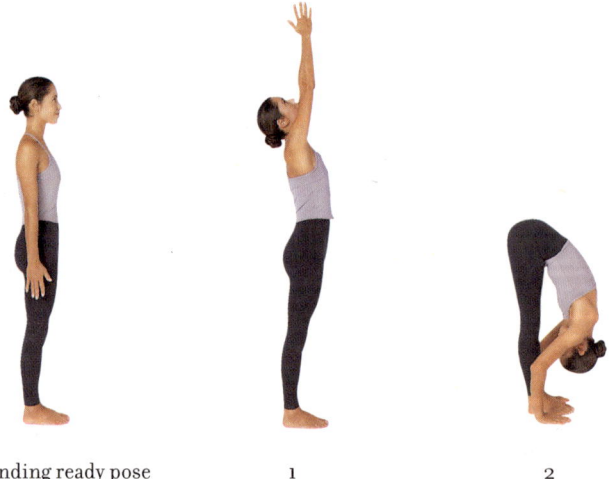

standing ready pose   1   2

2   Exhaling, fold forward from your hips, taking your head toward your shins and placing your hands on the floor on either side of your feet (or on your ankles or shins).

3   Inhaling, extend your spine and look up, straightening your arms but keeping your fingertips on the floor.

4   Exhaling, bend your knees and transfer your weight into your hands as you jump or step back (keeping your arms straight) into a raised press-up position. (Your legs should be straight and your shoulders should be above your wrists.) Continuing the movement bend your arms, lowering your body until your chin almost touches the floor. Keep your elbows pressed into your sides and look ahead.

(continued)

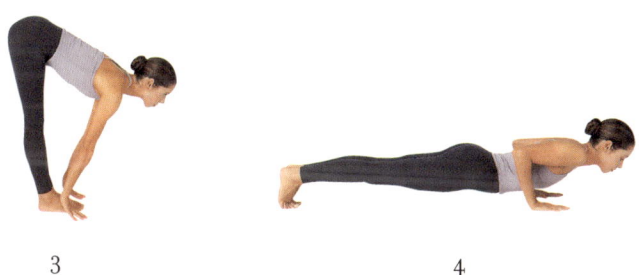

3   4

5   Inhaling, roll over your toes so that the tops of your feet are on the floor. Straighten your arms, bringing your chest through your hands. Keep your shoulders down and lift your chest. Raise your head and look up.

6   Exhaling, push back with your arms, roll back over your toes and lift your hips upward as you move into "downward dog" posture. Your hands should be shoulder-width apart, middle finger pointing forward, and your feet should be hip-width apart. Lengthen your spine and press down gently through your heels. Tuck in your chin and gaze toward your groin or navel. Hold this position for five full breaths (five inhalations and exhalations).

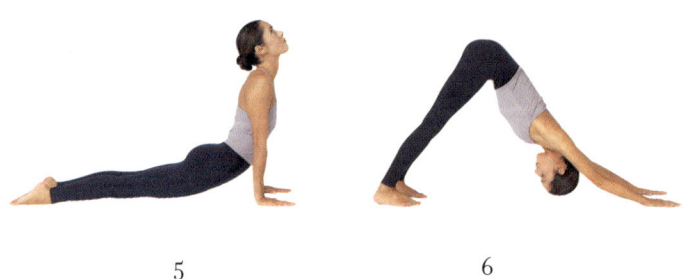

5   6

7 Inhaling, jump or walk your feet toward your hands.
   Keep your fingertips on the floor as you extend your
   spine and look up.

8 Exhaling, fold forward from your hips, taking your head
   toward your shins and releasing your spine.

9 Inhaling, raise your torso and arms, bringing your
   palms together above your head. Look up at your
   thumbs. Exhale, lowering your arms to your sides.
   Repeat the whole sequence five times.

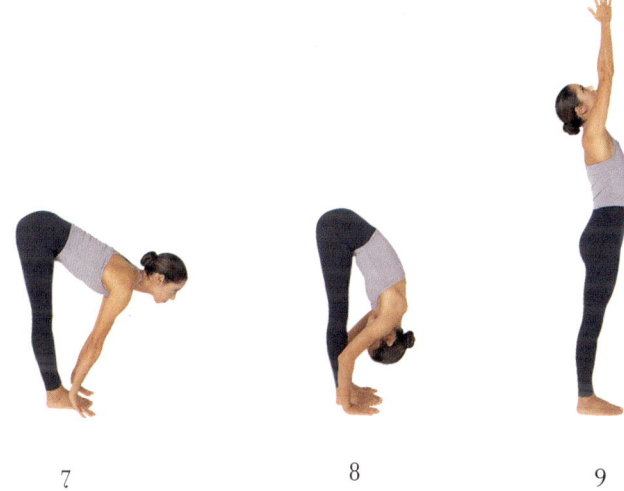

7   8   9

SUN SALUTATION B
Surya Namaskara B

1 Begin in standing ready pose. Inhaling, bend your knees and raise your arms above your head, bringing your palms together and looking up at your thumbs.

2 Exhaling, straighten your legs and fold forward from your hips, taking your head toward your shins and placing your hands on the floor on either side of your feet (or on your ankles or shins if necessary).

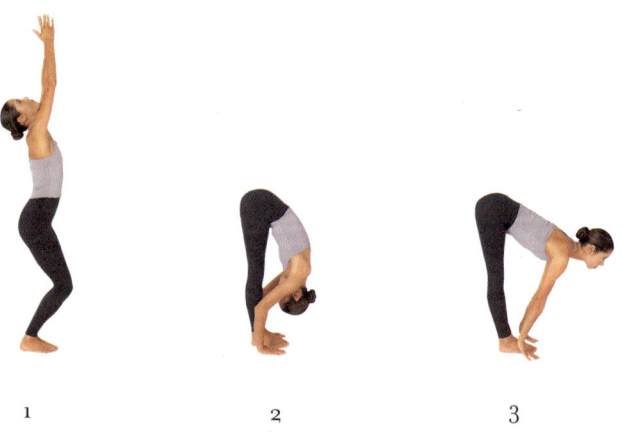

1   2   3

3 Inhaling, extend your spine as you look up, straightening your arms but keeping your hands down.

4 Exhaling, jump or step back into a raised press-up position. Then, bending your arms, lower your body until your chin almost touches the floor and look ahead.

5 Inhaling, roll over your toes and straighten your arms, bringing your chest through your hands. Keep your shoulders down, lift your chest and look up.

6 Exhaling, push back with your arms, roll back over your toes on to the soles of your feet and lift your hips toward the sky as you move into downward dog.

(continued)

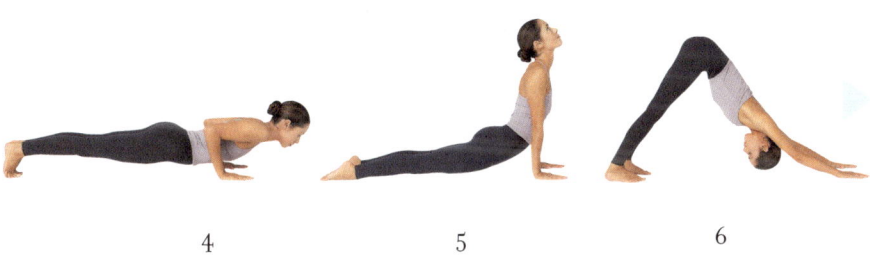

4   5   6

7 Inhaling, turn your left foot out 45° and step your right foot between your hands. Continuing the inhalation, raise your torso, lifting your arms above your head and bringing your palms together. Look up at your thumbs.

8 Exhaling, lower your hands to the floor and step your right foot back alongside your left, bringing you into a raised press-up position. Bending your arms, gently lower your body until your chin almost touches the floor and look ahead.

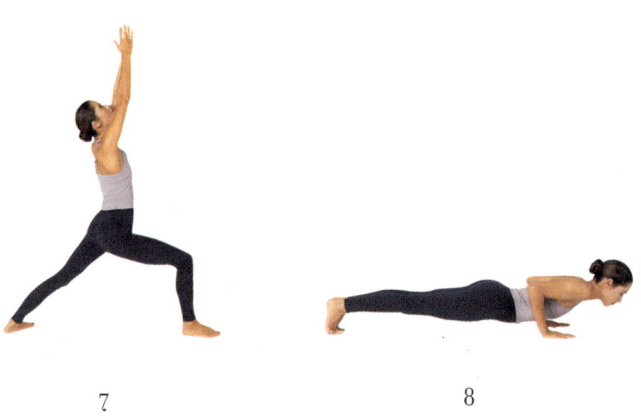

7   8

9   Inhaling, roll over your toes on to the tops of your feet and straighten your arms, bringing your chest through your hands. Keep your shoulders down, lift your chest and look up.

10 Exhaling, push back with your arms, roll back over your toes on to the soles of your feet and lift your hips toward the sky as you move into downward dog.

11 Inhaling, turn your right foot out 45°and step your left foot between your hands. Continuing the inhalation, raise your torso, lifting your hands above your head and bringing your palms together. Look up at your thumbs.

    (continued)

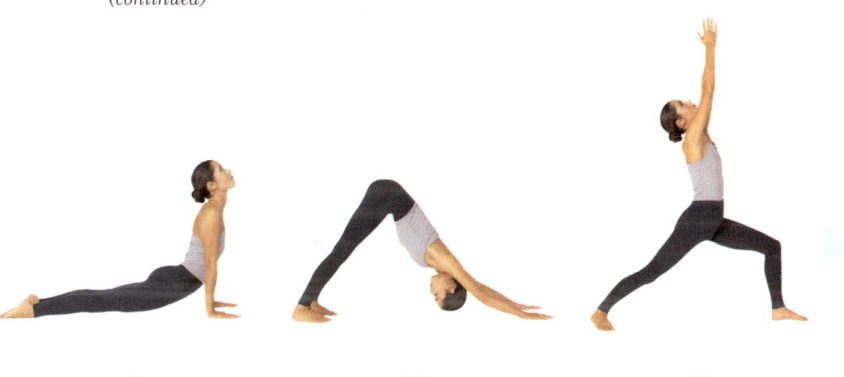

9   1O   11

12 Exhaling, lower your hands to the floor and step your left foot back alongside your right, bringing you into a raised press-up position. Bending your arms, lower your body until your chin almost touches the floor and look ahead.

13 Inhaling, roll over your toes and straighten your arms, bringing your chest through your hands. Keep your shoulders down, lift your chest and look up.

14 Exhaling, push back with your arms, roll back over your toes and lift your hips toward the sky as you move into downward dog. Lengthen your spine and press down through your heels. Tuck in your chin and gaze toward your groin or navel. Hold for five full breaths.

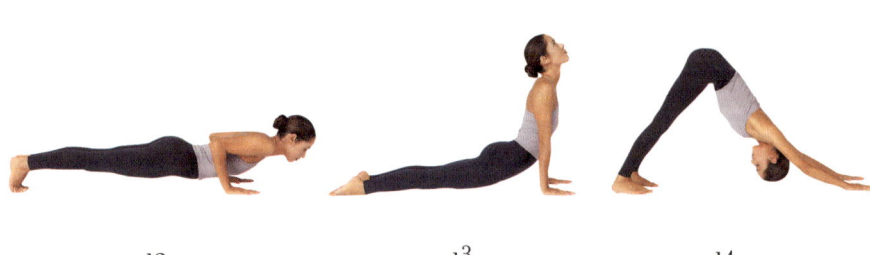

12   13   14

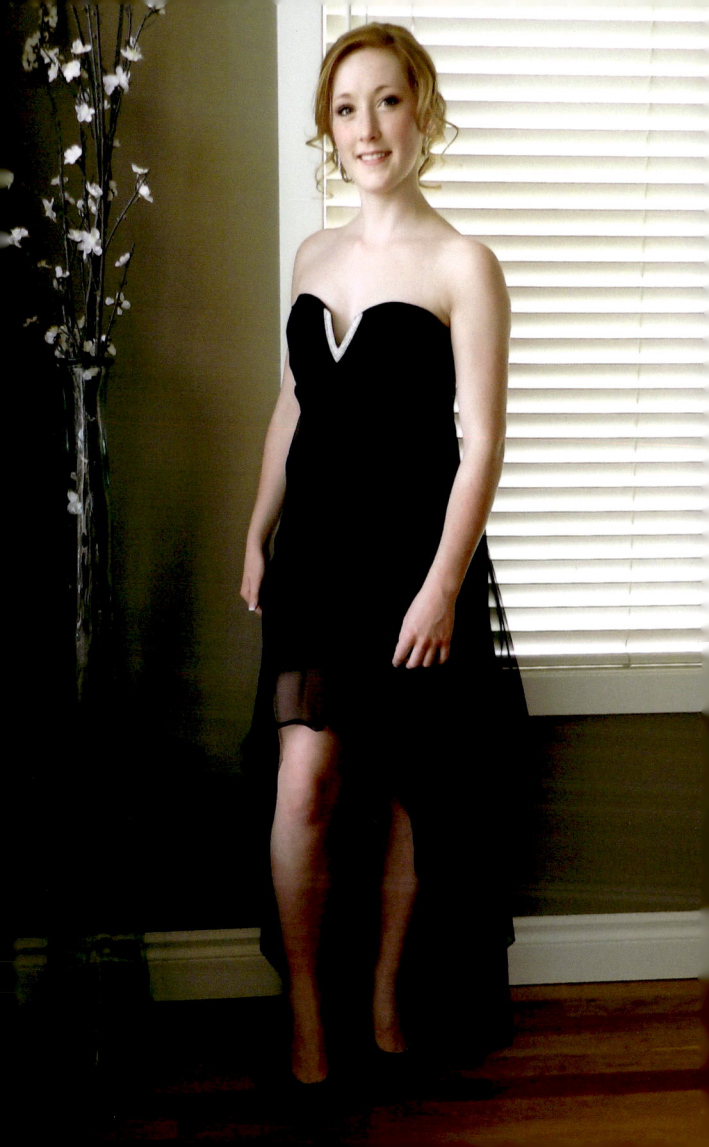

15 Inhaling, jump or walk your feet toward your hands, keeping your hands down as you extend your spine and look up.

16 Exhaling, fold forward from your hips, taking your head toward your shins and releasing your spine.

17 Inhaling, bend your knees before raising your torso and arms, bringing your palms together above your head. Look up at your thumbs. Exhaling, return to standing ready pose. Repeat the whole sequence five times.

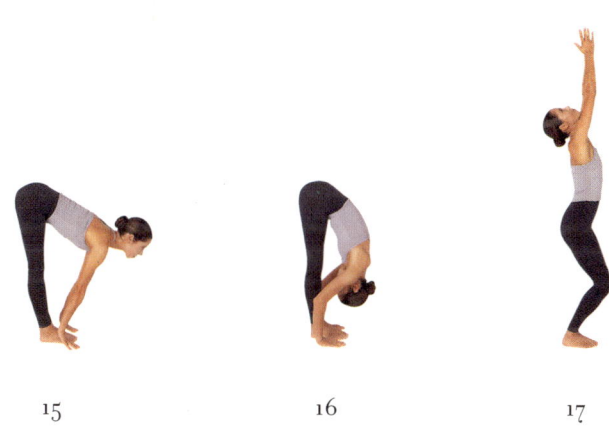

15   16   17

Body and breath, essence and energy are one:
when the body does not move, essence cannot flow;
when essence cannot flow, energy stagnates.

SUN SSU-MO, TANG-DYNASTY TAOIST PHYSICIAN
(581–681CE)

All living creatures depend on the breath
For it is the sustaining force of life itself,
Which determines how long all may live.
Those who revere breath as a gift from the Lord
Shall live to complete their full span of life.

TAITTIRIYA UPANISHAD (7TH CENTURY BCE)

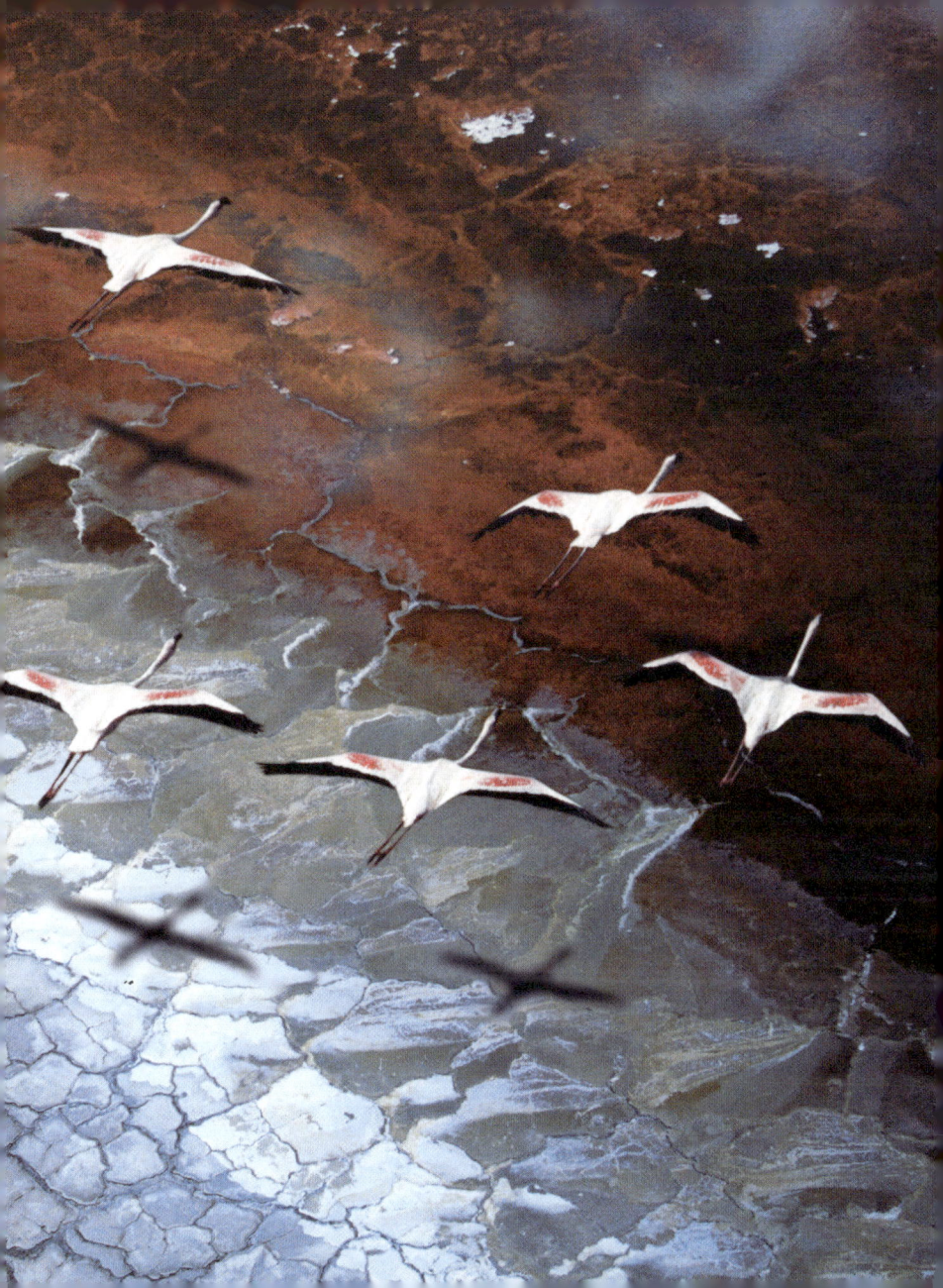

Chapter Three

the standing sequence

Once you have completed the sun salutations, your body should feel warm and you may even have begun to sweat. This is the ideal state for embarking upon the standing postures, which continue the process of opening up the body, loosening the joints and stretching out the muscles on a deeper level.

The standing postures encourage the development of strength and balance throughout the body. When practising these postures pay particular attention to your feet, for these are your foundation, your points of contact with the earth. Work on spreading the soles of your feet and splaying your toes to enlarge your base — this will improve your balance and the strength of your postures. If you find yourself off-balance, check the alignment of your feet and, if necessary, adjust your position accordingly.

Each of the postures in the Standing Sequence begins with *samasthiti*, the standing ready pose (see p.38). As you progress through the postures for the first time, focus initially on learning the positions and the movements leading into and out of each posture. When the sequence becomes more familiar, you can begin to link these movements with your *ujjayi* breathing, remembering that the breath should always lead the movement. The *bandhas* and *drishtis* will come with time, so try to be patient with yourself.

STANDING FORWARD BEND
Padangusthasana

1   Begin in standing ready pose. Inhaling, jump or step your feet hip-width apart. Exhaling, place your hands on your hips and relax your shoulders.

2   Inhaling, look up, lift and open your chest, lengthen the front of your body and draw your abdomen in. Exhaling, fold forward from your hips, lower your arms and hook around your big toes with the first two fingers of each hand. (Hold your ankles or shins if you cannot reach your toes.) Inhaling, pull against your grip and look up, extending your spine fully.

3   Exhaling, draw yourself down toward your legs, bending your elbows out to the sides. Look toward the tip of your nose and hold the position for five full breaths. To finish, inhaling, return to position 1. Exhaling, jump or step your feet back to the standing ready pose.

This posture stretches the spine and backs of the legs; massages the liver, spleen and kidneys; and reduces abdominal fat.

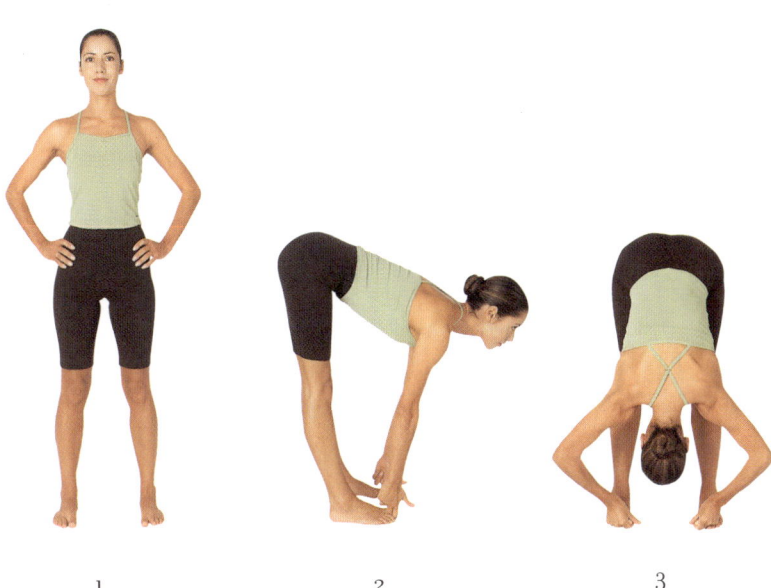

1

2

3

EXTENDED TRIANGLE
Utthita Trikonasana

1   Begin in standing ready pose. Inhaling, step to the right. Extend your arms horizontally out to the sides, palms down, and ensure that your feet line up beneath your elbows. Exhaling, turn your right foot out 90° and your left foot in 45°.

2   Inhaling, open your chest and lengthen your neck. Exhaling, fold sideways into your right hip, reaching down through your right arm to hook around your right big toe with your first two fingers. Extend up through your left arm, opening across your chest and shoulders. Turn your head to look up at your left thumb. Hold this position for five full breaths. Inhaling, return to position 1 and repeat the movement on your left side. To finish, inhaling, come up from the posture with your arms outstretched. Exhaling, return to standing ready pose.

This posture strengthens and tones the legs, hips and back as well as improving digestion and relieving breathing problems.

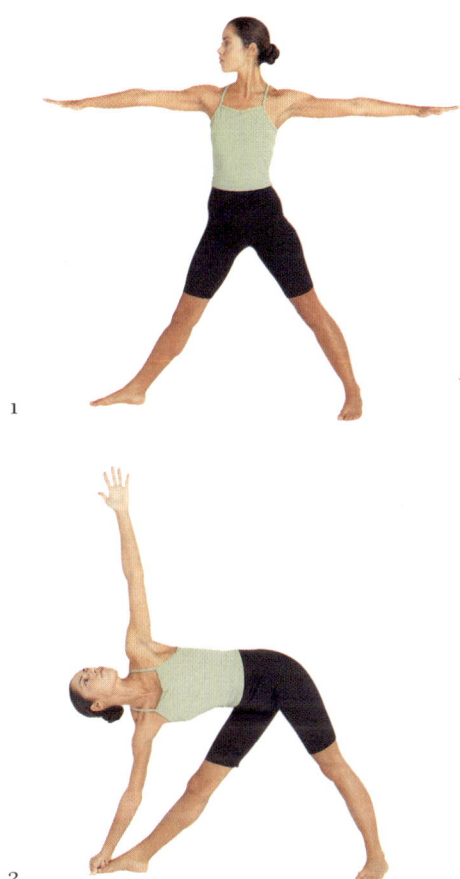

1

2

EXTENDED SIDE ANGLE
Utthita Parsvakonasana

1   Begin in standing ready pose. Inhaling, take a wide step to the right. Extend your arms horizontally out to the sides, palms down, and line up your feet beneath your wrists. Exhaling, turn your right foot out 90° and your left foot in 45°.

2   Inhaling, open your chest and shoulders. Exhaling, bend your right knee to form a right angle between your thigh and calf. Place your right hand outside your right foot, pressing your palm into the floor and your right knee into your armpit. Extend your left arm over your head and stretch down through your left foot. Look up at the extended hand and hold for five full breaths. Inhaling, return to position 1 and repeat the movement on your left side. To finish, inhaling, come up from the posture. Exhaling, return to standing ready pose.

This posture opens the ribcage, strengthens the arms, upper back, legs and hips, and improves digestion and breathing.

EXTENDED SIDE ANGLE

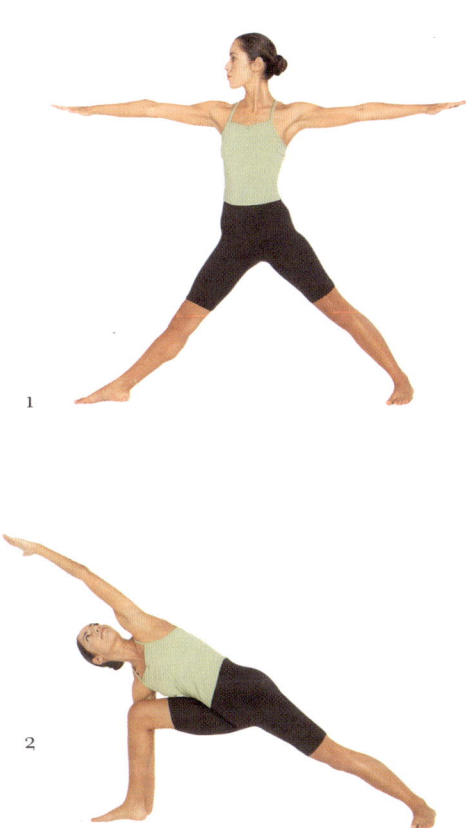

1

2

57

FEET SPREAD INSIDE STRETCH
Prasarita Padottanasana

1 Begin in standing ready pose. Inhaling, take a wide step to the right. Extend your arms horizontally out to the sides and line up your feet beneath your wrists, with your heels in line and the outsides of your feet parallel.

2 Exhaling, lower your hands to your hips.

3 Inhaling, open your chest and look up. Exhaling, fold forward and place your hands on the floor, shoulder-width apart, with your elbows tucked in. Inhaling, straighten your arms, extend the spine and look up.

4 Exhaling, lower your torso, taking your head toward the floor and allowing your arms to bend. Look toward the tip of your nose and hold for five full breaths. To finish, inhaling, straighten your arms and look up. Exhaling, place your hands on your hips. Inhaling, come up to position 2. Exhaling, return to standing ready pose.

This posture lengthens the inner thighs, stimulates the pelvic organs and encourages the flow of blood to the brain.

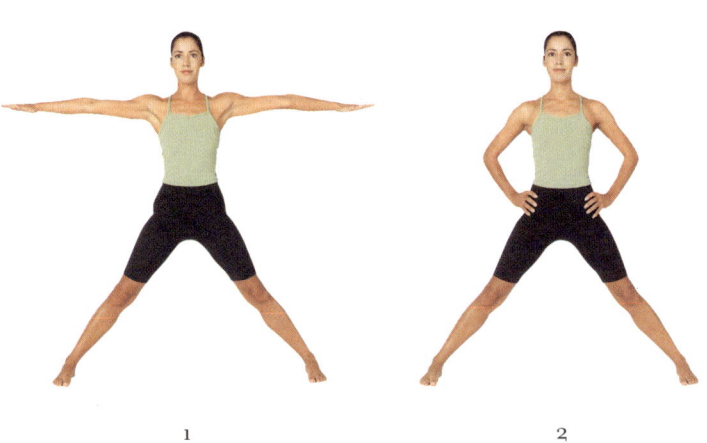

1

2

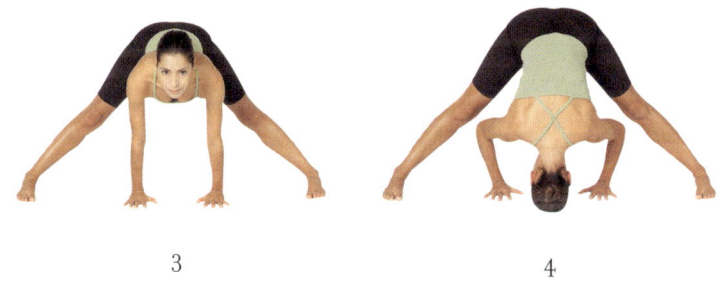

3

4

SIDE FORWARD STRETCH
Parsvottanasana

1   Begin in standing ready pose. Inhaling, step to the right. Extend your arms horizontally to the sides, palms down, and line up your feet roughly beneath your elbows. Exhaling, turn your right foot out 90° and your left foot in 45°. Turning to face your right foot, bring your hips square and join your hands behind your back in prayer position. Inhaling, press your palms together, arch your spine, open your chest and look up.

2   Exhaling, fold forward toward your right shin, leading with your chin. (If necessary bend your right knee slightly.) Look toward your right big toe and hold this position for five full breaths. Inhaling, return to position 1 and repeat the movement on your left side. To finish come up on the sixth inhalation and bring your feet parallel. Exhaling, return to standing ready pose.

This posture opens the hips, improves balance, tones the abdomen and clears the digestive and respiratory tracts.

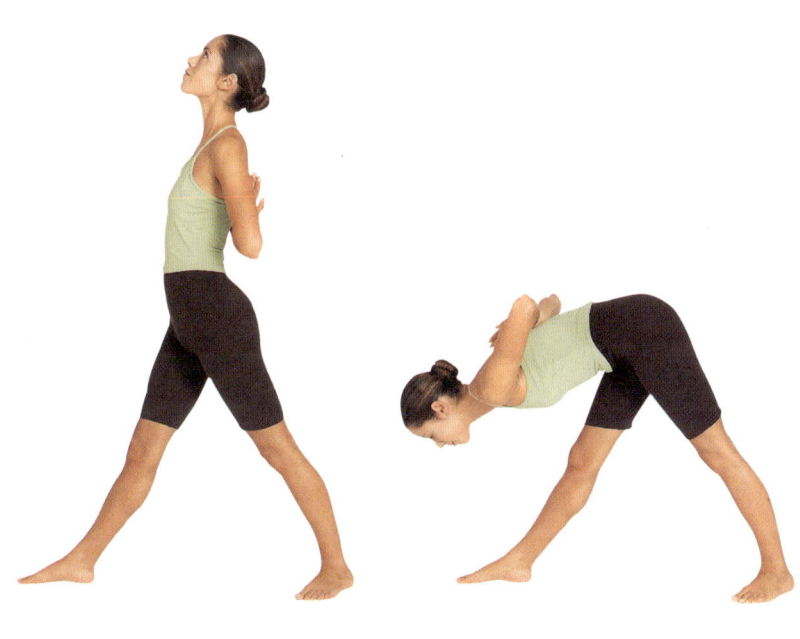

1

2

EXTENDED STANDING LEG RAISES
Utthita Hasta Padangusthasana

1   Begin in standing ready pose. Inhaling, bend and raise your right leg, hooking around your big toe with the first two fingers of your right hand. Place your left hand on your left hip and grip firmly.

2   Exhaling, extend your right leg out as straight as possible in front of you, while maintaining your grip on your big toe. Look at the held toe or focus on a fixed point straight ahead of you to help you maintain your balance. Hold this position for five full breaths.

3   Inhaling, lift and open your chest. Exhaling, take your right leg out to the right. Turn your head to look over your left shoulder and focus on a fixed point. Hold the posture for five full breaths. Inhaling, return to position 2. Exhaling, release your grip and return to standing ready pose. Repeat the exercise with your left leg.

This posture increases the flexibility of the hips, strengthens the legs and stimulates the kidneys and digestive system.

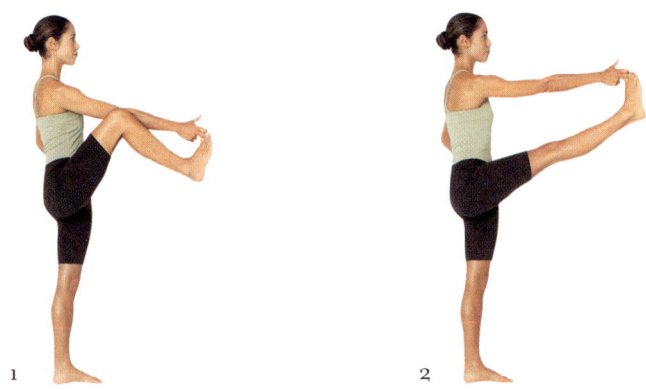

1

2

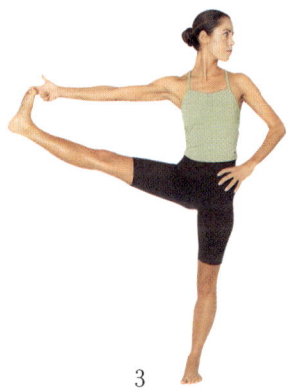

3

TREE POSE
Vrkshasana

1 Begin in standing ready pose. Inhaling, shift your weight on to your left leg. Keeping your left leg straight, lift your right leg, taking hold of your right ankle with your right hand. Exhaling, place the sole of your right foot on the inside of your left thigh, bringing the heel as close to your groin as possible. Press the thigh and foot together while drawing your right knee back. Focus ahead on a fixed point to maintain balance.

2 Inhaling, lift your chest, roll your shoulders back and extend upward through your spine. Exhaling, bring your hands into prayer position in front of your chest. Look at the tip of your nose or focus on a fixed point ahead. Hold this position for five full breaths. Inhaling, lift the foot off the thigh. Exhaling, return to standing ready pose. Repeat the exercise on the left side.

This posture strengthens the feet and ankles, opens the hips, increases knee flexibility and improves balance and focus.

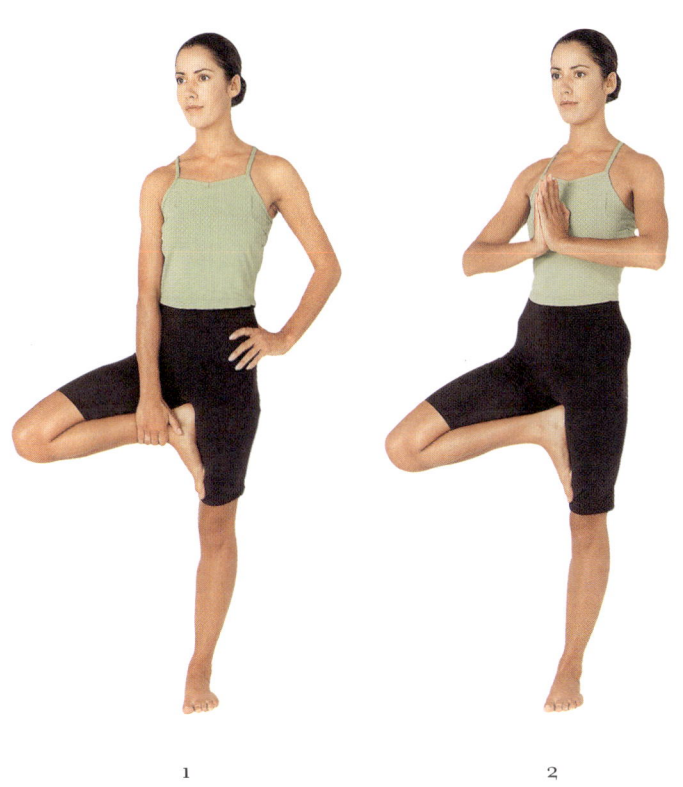

1   2

WARRIOR SEQUENCE
Virabhadrasana

The warrior sequence marks the end of the standing postures and provides a smooth transition into the floor postures. The sequence improves overall strength, flexibility and stamina, realigns the spine, opens the ribcage, stretches the inner thighs and tones the buttocks and abdominals.

1   Starting from standing ready pose, perform steps 1–6 of sun salutation A (see pp.38–41). Hold position 6 (down-ward dog) for one full breath.

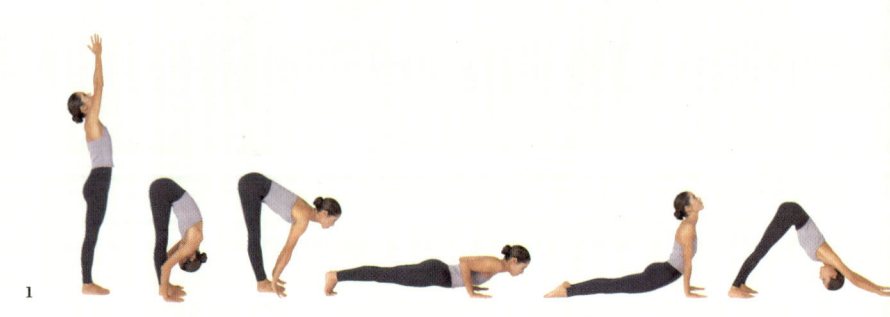

1

2   Inhaling, bend your knees and jump your feet toward your hands. Keeping your feet together and your knees bent, tuck in your tailbone as you sit down into the posture. Raise your arms, bringing your palms together above your head. Look up toward your thumbs and hold this position for five full breaths.

(continued)

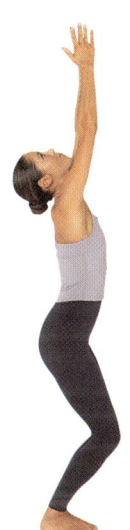

2

3 Inhaling, straighten your legs, reaching up with your hands as you return to position 1 of sun salutation A. Move through steps 1–6 of sun salutation A, remaining in position 6 (downward dog) for one full breath.

4 Inhaling, turn your left foot out 45° and step your right foot toward your hands. Continuing the inhalation, bend your right knee to form a right angle between your thigh and calf, adjusting your feet if necessary. As you do so raise your torso, bringing your palms together above your head. Ensure that your back leg is straight and your back foot is flat on the floor. Look up at your thumbs. Hold the position for five full breaths.

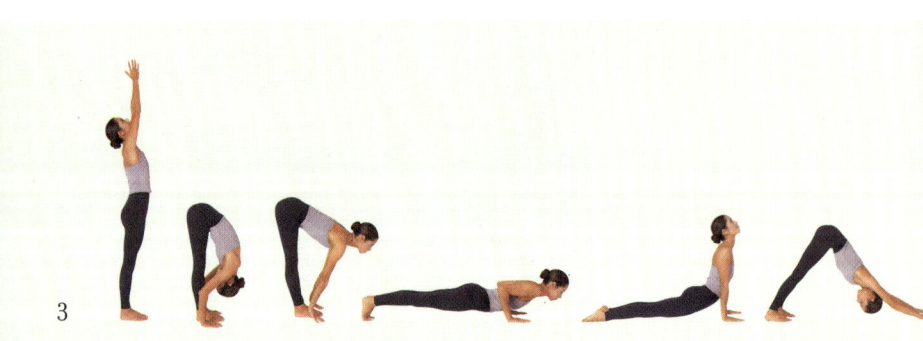

3

5   Inhaling, keep your arms above your head with the palms pressed together as you straighten your right leg, pivot your left foot out and your right foot in, and rotate your body around to face the opposite direction. Exhaling, bend your left knee to form a right angle between your thigh and calf. Adjust the space between your feet if necessary and ensure that your back leg is straight and your back foot is flat on the floor. Look up at your thumbs. Hold the position for five full breaths.

(continued)

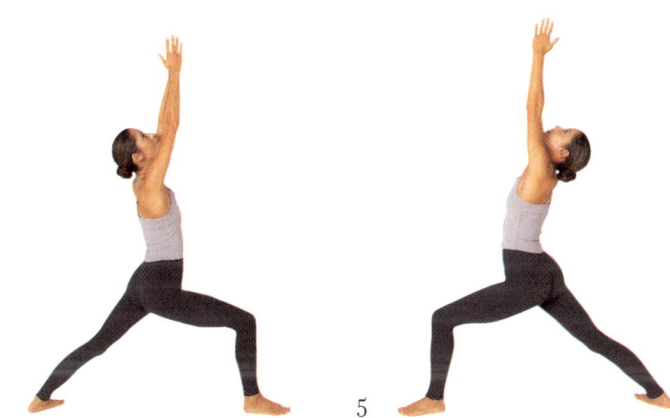

4   5

6   Exhaling, lower your arms until they extend out horizontally over your legs, palms down. Stretch out through
your fingers, opening your chest and shoulders. Look
toward the middle finger of your left hand. Hold the
position for five full breaths.

7   Inhaling, keep your arms parallel to the floor as you
straighten your left leg, pivoting your right foot out and
your left foot in. As you do so rotate your body round to
face the opposite direction. Exhaling, bend your right
knee to form a right angle between your thigh and calf.

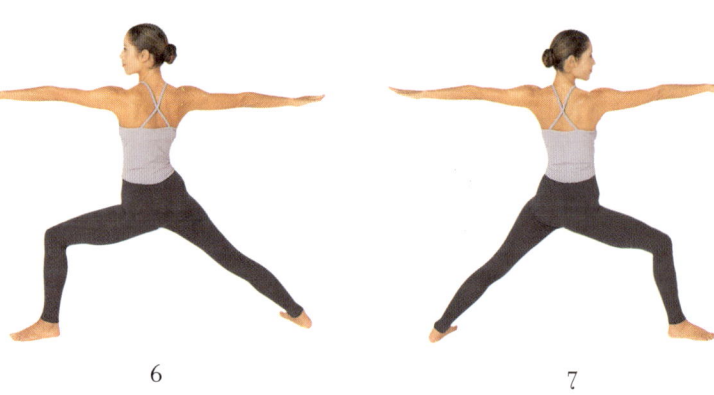

6   7

Adjust the space between your feet if necessary and ensure that your back leg is straight and your back foot is flat on the floor. Look toward the middle finger of your right hand. Hold the position for five full breaths.

8   Inhaling, move your left arm round so that it is next to your right. Exhaling, take your hands to the floor, on either side of your right foot, and step back into a raised press-up position. Lower yourself into position 4 of sun salutation A. Repeat steps 4–9 of sun salutation A, holding position 6 (downward dog) for one full breath.

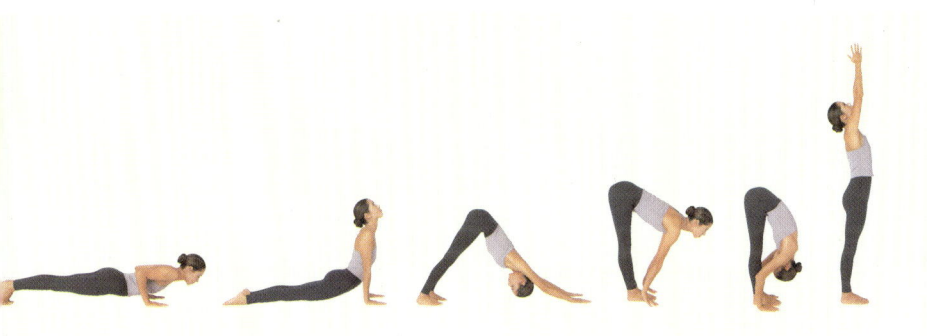

8

Away from the chatter of the senses
From the restless wanderings of the mind
There is a quiet pool of stillness.
The wise call this stillness the highest state of being.
It is the place where we find unity.

Never to become separate again.

KATHA UPANISHAD (5TH CENTURY BCE)

It has its roots in the worlds above
And its branches on earth below.
It is the Tree of all Eternity.
Its pure root is Brahman – the Immortal Giver of Life
Whom none can transcend.

KATHA UPANISHAD (5TH CENTURY BCE)

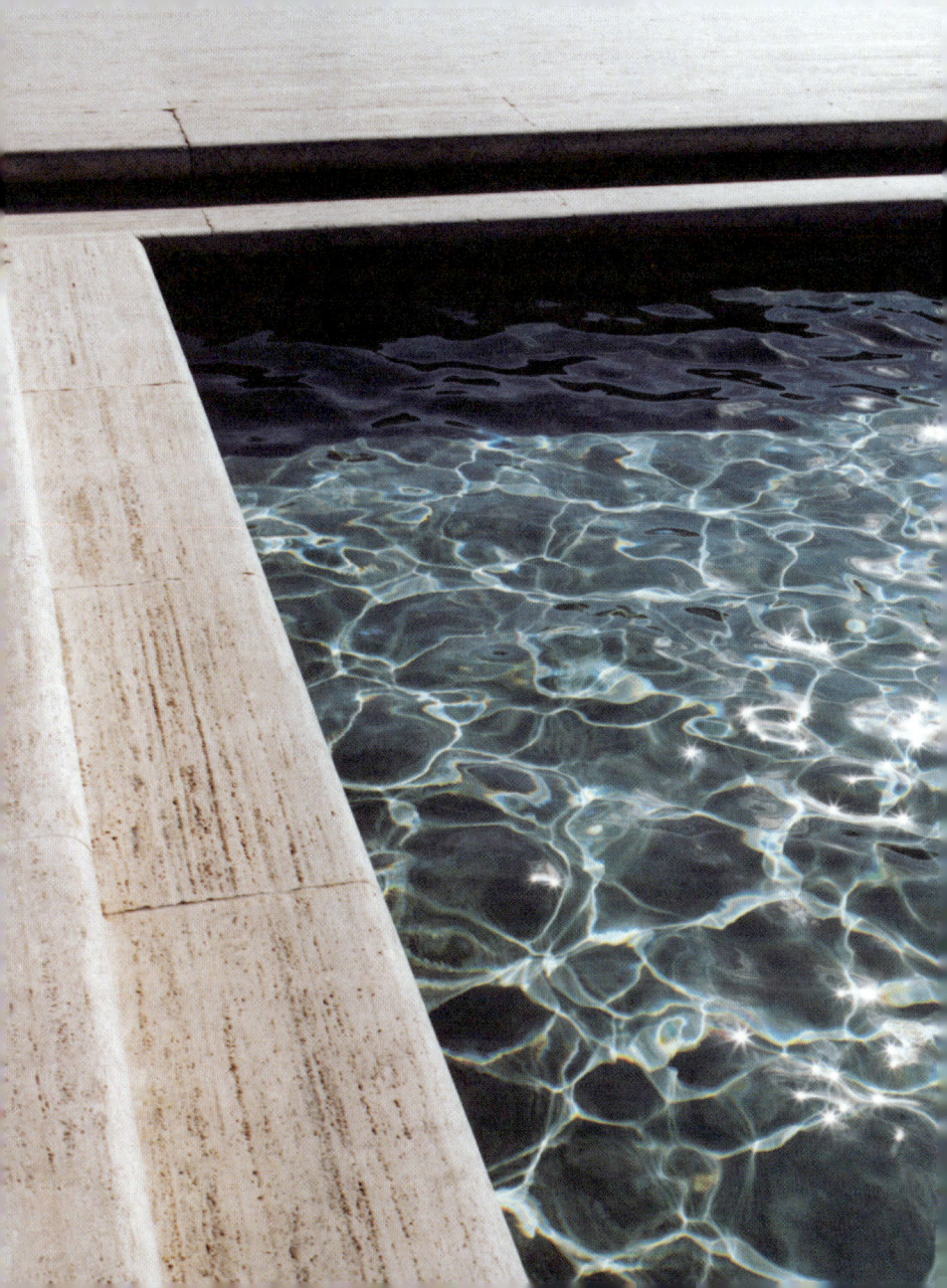

Chapter Four

the floor sequence

The floor postures of the Primary Series extend the process that is begun in the Standing Sequence. We explore a new relationship with our foundation as our principal points of contact with the floor shift from our feet to our buttocks and hands, which provide a broader base and a lower centre of gravity. The result is a greater sense of stability that allows us to deepen our focus on the breath and enhance our internal awareness. The floor postures also bring us into greater contact with the root *chakra* (see pp.16–19), which has a grounding effect on our emotions.

A number of the postures in this chapter are forward bends, where the torso bends over the legs.

These serve to lengthen the spine, improving flexibility and opening the vertebrae, as well as stretching and lengthening the hamstrings. To counterbalance these postures the sequence also includes more open poses that flex the spine in the opposite direction.

A half-*vinyasa* (see pp.76–7) is performed between each posture: this chapter presents a modified version that is suitable for beginners. As well as linking the postures, half-*vinyasas* sustain the internal heat generated during the earlier sequences. They also rebalance and centre our bodies between postures, and work on our upper body and abdominal strength – helping us to develop greater internal support.

HALF-VINYASA

1 Begin in sitting ready pose with your legs straight out in front of you, feet together, hands flat on the floor just behind your hips. Inhaling, cross your legs, bringing your feet as close to your buttocks as possible. Place your palms on the floor ahead of your feet, slightly more than shoulder-width apart with the fingers pointing forward.

2 Pressing down through your hands, roll forward over your ankles, lifting your buttocks off the floor.

3 Maintaining the lift during the exhalation, shift your weight forward and jump your legs backward into a raised press-up position. Bending your arms, lower your body until your chin almost touches the floor.

4 Inhaling, roll over your toes, straighten your arms, bring your chest through your arms and look up.

5 Exhaling, push back with your arms into downward dog. Hold this position for one full breath. Inhaling, return to position 2 by jumping your feet toward your hands, crossing your ankles as you land. Exhaling, straighten your legs in preparation for the next floor posture.

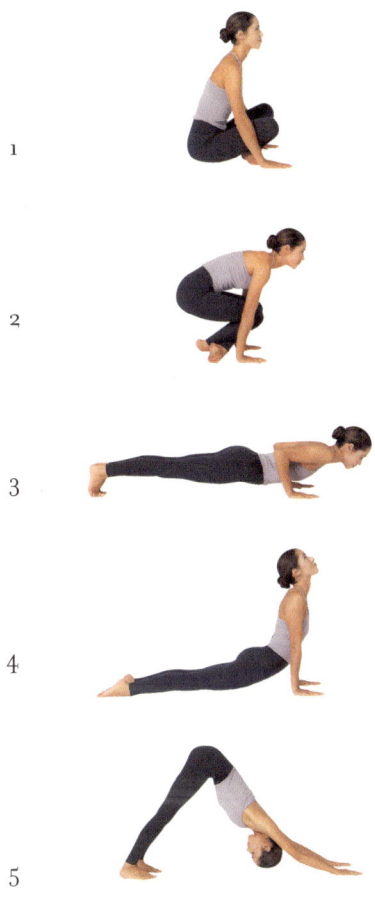

1

2

3

4

5

STAFF POSTURE/SEATED FORWARD BEND
Dandasana/Paschimattanasana

1 Adopt sitting ready pose with your legs straight out in front of you, feet together, and your hands flat on the floor, just behind your hips, fingers pointing forward. Inhaling, lift your chest and draw your shoulders back. Exhaling, lower your chin and flex your ankles. Look at your toes or your nose. Hold for five full breaths.

2 Inhaling, lift your chin, extend up through your spine and draw in your abdomen. Exhaling, reach forward and hook around your two big toes with the first two fingers of each hand. Inhaling, lengthen your spine and look up.

3 Exhaling, use your arms to draw yourself forward over your legs. Bend your elbows out to the sides as you extend your chin toward your shins. Look at your toes and hold for five full breaths. Inhaling, return to position 1. After exhaling perform a half-*vinyasa*.

This posture stretches the spine and hamstrings, massages the internal organs and strengthens the heart.

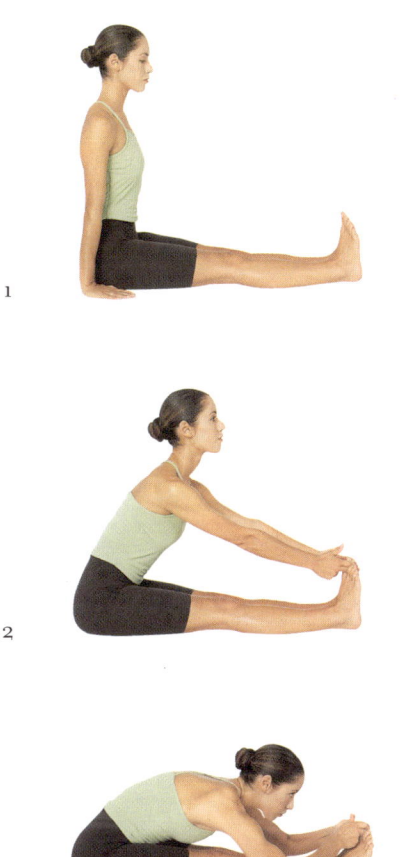

1

2

3

INCLINED BACK LIFT
Purvattanasana

1 Begin in sitting ready pose, pressing your palms into the floor and lifting your chest as you inhale. Exhaling, place your hands between 20 and 30 cm (7.9–11.8 in) behind your hips, shoulder-width apart with the fingers pointing forward.

2 Inhaling, raise your hips, keeping the legs and feet together. Gently allow your head to relax backward, without shortening your neck. Push the soles of your feet into the floor to help keep your legs straight and lift your pelvis. Push down through your hands, rolling your shoulders back as you lift and open your chest. Look toward your "third eye" (see p.27) and hold the position for five full breaths. Inhaling, lift your head. Exhaling, lower your hips to the floor and release your arms. Now perform a half-*vinyasa*.

This posture strengthens the arms, shoulders and abdomen, opens the ribcage and relaxes the nervous system.

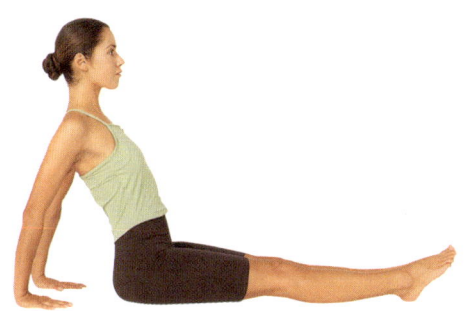

1

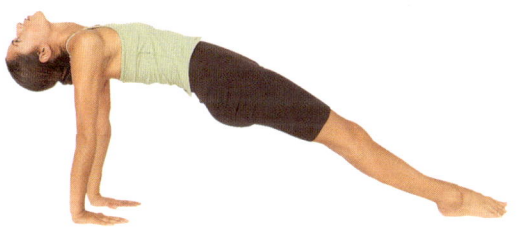

2

HEAD-TO-KNEE POSTURE
Janu Sirsasana

1 Begin in sitting ready pose. Inhaling, lift and bend your right leg, cupping the ankle in your left hand. Exhaling, bring your heel to your groin so that the sole of your foot runs along the inside of your left thigh. Your right knee should point out to the side at 90°, with the knee as close to the floor as possible.

2 Inhaling, fold forward over your left leg, taking hold of your left foot (or shin) with both hands. Pull against your grip, extend through your spine and look up.

3 Exhaling, bring your chest closer to your knee and your chin to your shin. Look at the toes of your left foot and hold the position for five full breaths. To finish, inhaling, raise your head and extend your spine. Exhaling, release your hands and straighten your legs. Repeat the exercise on your left side, then perform a half-*vinyasa*.

This posture stretches the legs; opens the lower back, hips and knees; and stimulates the circulation and urinary systems.

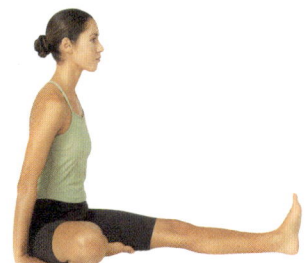

1

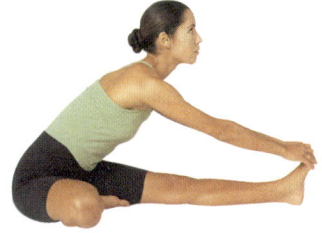

2

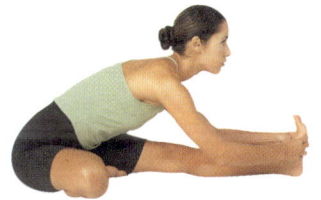

3

SON OF BRAHMA POSTURE
Marichyasana

1 Begin in sitting ready pose. Exhaling, bend your right knee, bringing your right foot toward your right hip. Align the outside of your right heel with the outside of your right buttock and place your left hand flat on the floor by your left hip. Inhaling, extend your right arm above your head, lengthen your abdomen and look up.

2 Exhaling, fold forward, wrap your right arm around your right leg and bring your hands together behind you. Aim to clasp your left wrist with your right hand. Inhaling, lengthen through your spine and look up.

3 Exhaling, bring your chest toward your left knee. Look at the toes of your left foot and hold for five full breaths. To finish, inhaling, extend your spine and look up. Exhaling, release the posture. Repeat the exercise on your left side, then perform a half-*vinyasa*.

This posture relieves tension in the lower back, cleanses the kidneys, regulates the digestion and eases constipation.

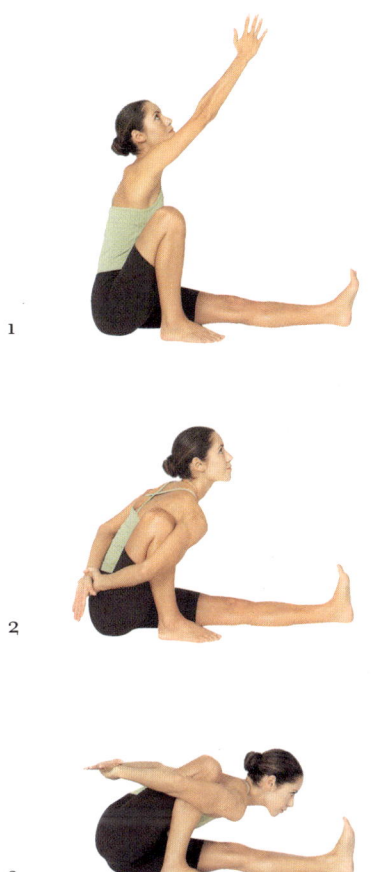

1

2

3

BOAT POSTURE
Navasana

1 Begin in sitting ready pose. Inhaling, lean back and lift your legs in front of you, keeping your feet together, toes pointed and legs straight (bend your knees if necessary). Bring your arms parallel to the floor, palms facing each other. Extend through your fingers, lift your chest and roll your shoulders back. Look at your toes. Hold for five full breaths.

2 Inhaling, place your hands flat on the floor, on either side of your hips with the fingers pointing forward. Exhaling, cross your legs at the ankles and bring your knees toward your chest. Pushing down through your hands, draw in your abdomen, shorten your torso and lift your body off the floor. Inhaling, lower your body to the floor and return to position 1. Repeat this exercise three to five times before performing a half-*vinyasa*.

This posture strengthens the abdominals and lower back, and stimulates the visceral organs — in particular the intestines.

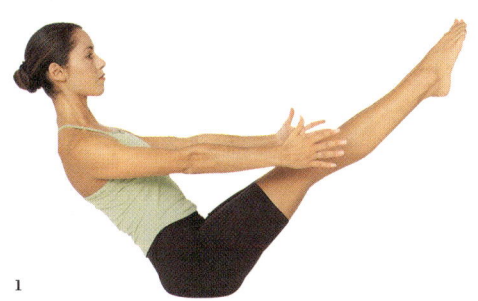

1

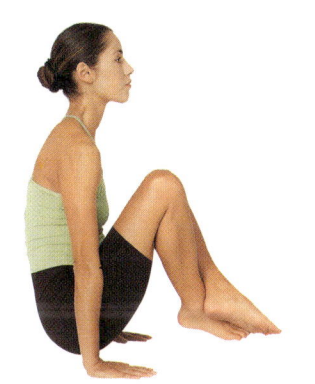

2

BOUND ANGLE POSTURE
Baddha Konasana

1 Begin in sitting ready pose. Exhaling, bring both feet in toward your groin with your soles together. Clasp your feet in your hands, relax the muscles in your hips and groin, and allow your knees to drop toward the floor.

2 Inhaling, press your thumbs into your soles just below the ball of each foot and open out your feet, exposing the soles. Use the rotation of your feet to lower your knees further. Lift your chest, roll your shoulders back and lengthen your spine.

3 Exhaling, fold forward over your feet, keeping your spine lengthened and chest lifted. Bend your elbows, using your forearms to place a downward pressure on your thighs. Look at the tip of your nose and hold for five full breaths. Inhaling, sit upright. Exhaling, release the posture before performing a half-*vinyasa*.

This posture opens the hips, stretches the inner thighs, strengthens the back and improves pelvic circulation.

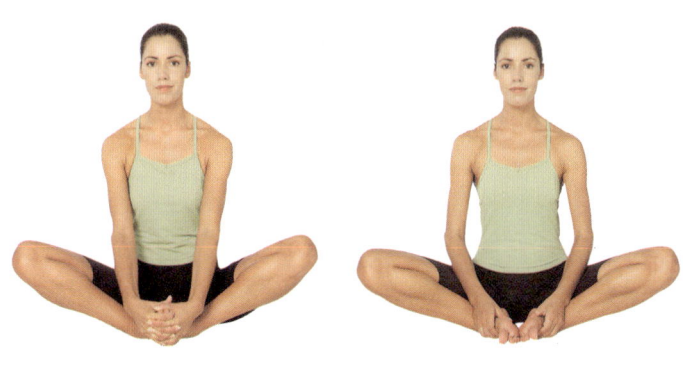

1   2

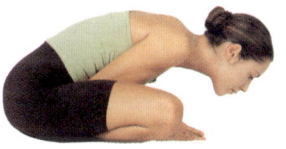

3

BRIDGE POSTURE
Setu Bandhasana

1 Begin in sitting ready pose. Exhaling, lie flat on your back, bending your knees and placing your feet flat on the floor as close to your buttocks as possible. Keeping your heels together, turn out your feet, allowing your knees to move apart while maintaining contact between the floor and the soles of your feet.

2 Inhaling, place your palms on the floor, thumbs tucked beneath your buttocks. Bend your arms and lift your torso, supporting your body on your forearms. Arch your back and roll your head back on to the floor.

3 Exhaling, fold your arms across your chest, placing a hand on each shoulder. Distribute your weight between your head, buttocks and feet. Look at the tip of your nose and hold for five full breaths. Inhaling, place your fore-arms on the floor and lift your head. Exhaling, return to sitting ready pose and perform a half-*vinyasa*.

This posture opens the chest, increasing breathing capacity.

BRIDGE POSTURE

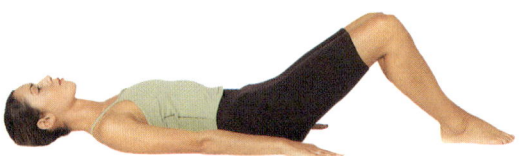

1

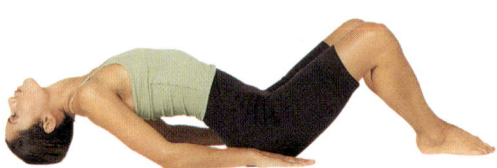

2

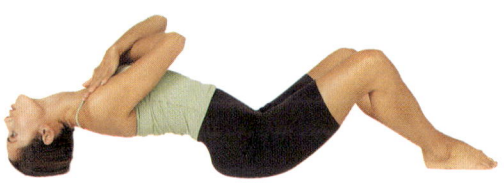

3

ELEVATED UPWARD BOW
Urdhva Dhanurasana

1 Begin in sitting ready pose. Exhaling, lie flat on your back with your arms by your sides. Bend your knees, placing your feet close to your buttocks, flat on the floor, slightly wider than hip-width apart.

2 Inhaling, grip your ankles with your hands and push upward with your hips, allowing your back to curve. Bear your weight through your shoulders rather than through your neck. Look at the tip of your nose and hold for five full breaths and a sixth inhalation. During the sixth exhalation lower yourself slowly to the floor. Repeat this exercise three times. When you have finished perform seated forward bend (see pp.78–9), holding the posture for ten full breaths. Then perform a half-*vinyasa*.

This energizing posture develops the strength and flexibility of the whole body, particularly the spine, legs, buttocks, arms, shoulders and upper back. It also stretches the front of the legs and abdomen, and opens out the chest and shoulders.

ELEVATED UPWARD BOW

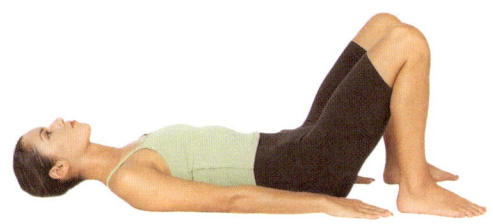

1

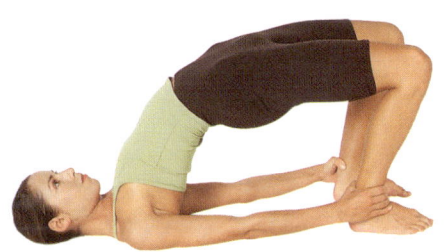

2

Withdraw in meditation from the pleasures
of sense as a tortoise withdraws its limbs.
Through this will you find peace.

BHAGAVAD GITA (6TH CENTURY BCE)

Compose yourself in stillness
Draw your attention inward
And devote your consciousness to the Self.
For the wisdom you seek lies within.

BHAGAVAD GITA (6TH CENTURY BCE)

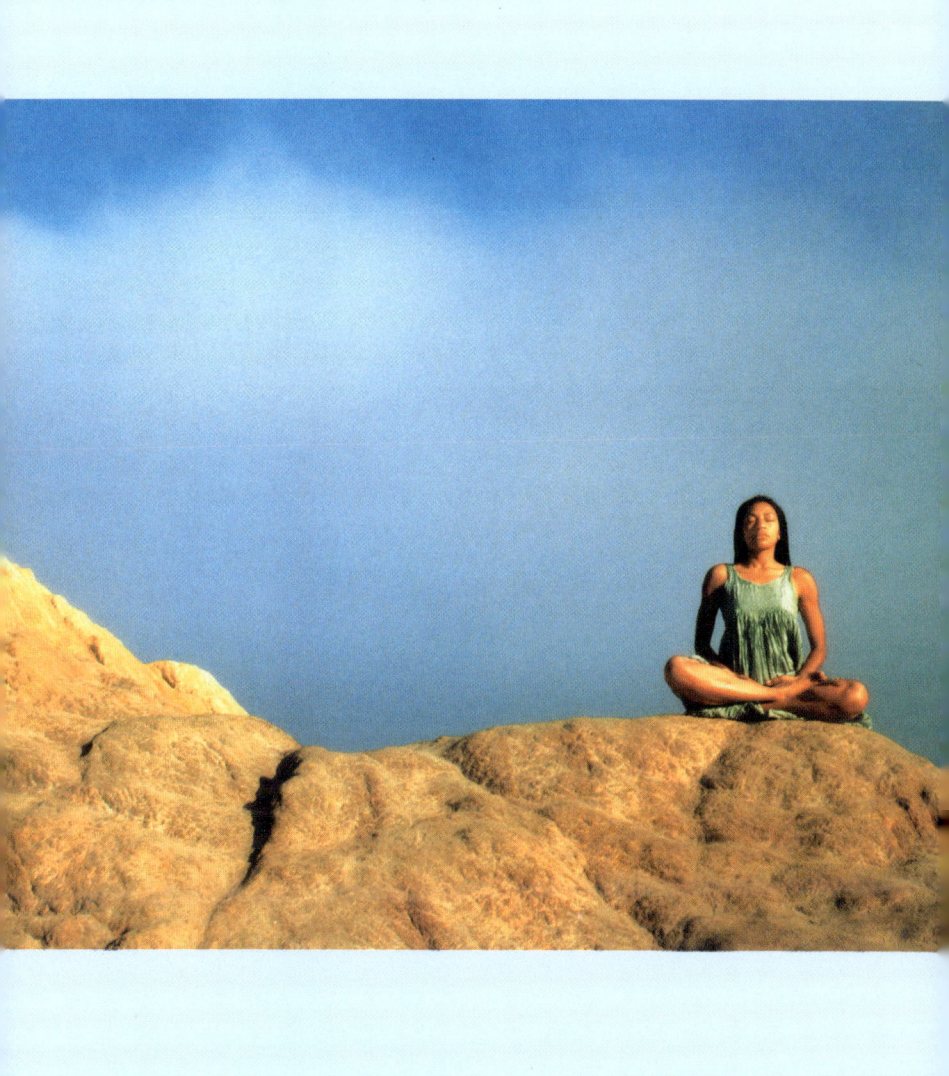

the finishing sequence

The Finishing Sequence is a vital component of any Ashtanga practice, however short, and should be neither rushed nor skipped. The sequence is composed of a number of inverted postures (in which the body is turned upside-down) together with some balancing counterposes. Inverting the body results in an increased supply of oxygenated blood to the head. This enhances brain function, improving our sensory awareness and enabling us to think more clearly and effectively, with greater concentration.

Each posture is held for longer than in previous sequences and the rate of the *ujjayi* breathing is slowed. This serves to return the body to a state of internal equilibrium as the muscles relax, cellular respiration slows, the uptake of oxygen from the blood decreases, the heart rate lowers and the body temperature begins to cool.

Throughout the sequence you should maintain *ujjayi* breathing. However, as you progress through the postures allow each breath to become longer and more relaxed, until finally you resume normal breathing in corpse posture (see p.108).

The postures of the Finishing Sequence should leave you feeling relaxed and refreshed. They are perfect for doing either on their own or together with some sun salutations after a busy day at work.

SHOULDERSTAND/PLOUGH POSTURE
Salamba Sarvangasana/Halasana

1 Exhaling, lie down with your arms by your sides. After five long breaths, inhale as you press your arms into the floor, lift your legs and roll up on to your shoulders.

2 Bend your elbows and use your hands to support your back. When you feel stable straighten your legs, pointing up through your toes and drawing in your abdomen to support your back. Look toward your toes or the tip of your nose and hold the position for ten long breaths.

3 Exhaling, bring your feet to the floor behind you, keeping your back upright and legs straight. Then place your arms flat on the floor and interlock your hands. Look toward your abdomen or the tip of your nose. Hold this position for ten long breaths. Inhaling, separate your hands, using them for support as you return your legs to position 1. Exhaling, roll out of the posture.

This rejuvenating posture stretches and strengthens the upper body, stimulates circulation and improves digestion.

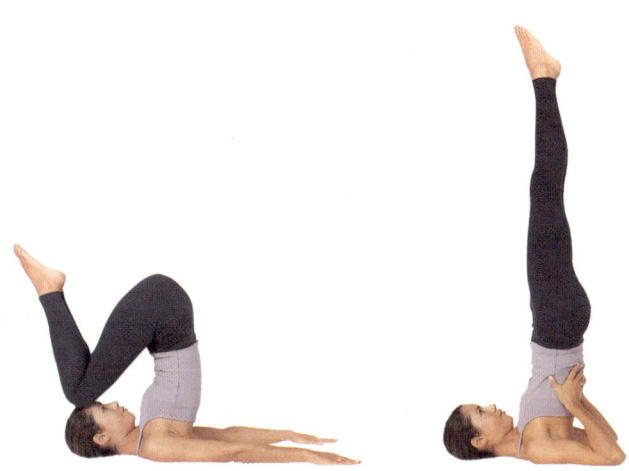

1

2

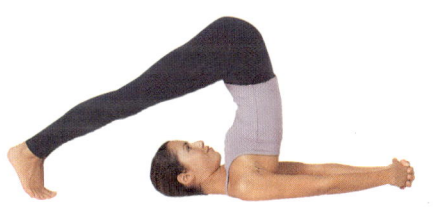

3

FISH POSTURE/EXTENDED LEG POSTURE
Matsyasana/Uttanapadasana

1 Begin by lying on your back, legs outstretched. Inhaling, place your hands next to your buttocks, bend your elbows and raise your upper body on to your forearms.

2 Exhaling, arch backward, allowing your head to relax back on to the floor. Open your chest, lengthen through your abdomen and point your toes. Look toward your "third eye" and hold the posture for ten long breaths.

3 Supporting your weight with your head and lower body, release your arms as you exhale, extending them over your torso with the palms together. Keeping your legs straight and your feet together, lift them off the floor, pointing your fingers toward your feet. Look at the tip of your nose and hold for ten long breaths. Inhaling, return your forearms to the floor and raise your head. Exhaling, lower your torso and legs to the floor.

A counterpose to shoulderstand, this posture relieves upper back tension and opens the chest, shoulders and neck.

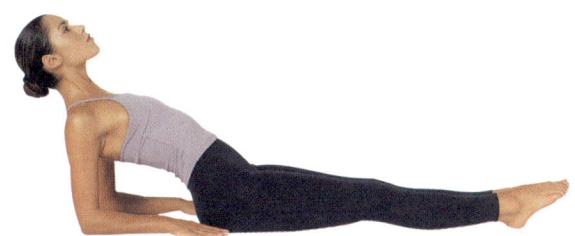

1

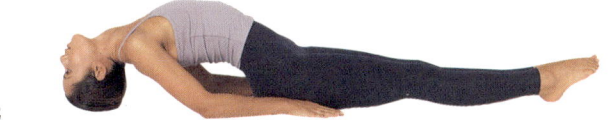

2

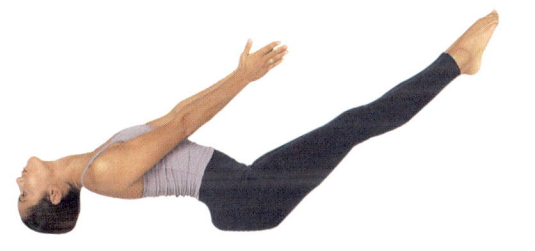

3

HEADSTAND
Shirhsasana

1 Inhaling, kneel down. Place your forearms on the floor in front of you and touch each elbow with the fingertips of the opposite hand. Exhaling, without moving your elbows, rotate your forearms outward and interlock your fingers to form a triangle-shaped foundation. Place the crown of your head on the floor between them. Inhaling, straighten your legs, lifting your hips upward.

2 Exhaling, walk your feet toward your head. Inhaling, support your weight through your arms and shoulders as you lift your feet off the floor, bending your knees.

3 When you feel confident, straighten your legs as you exhale, pointing your toes, drawing in your abdomen and pushing down through your forearms. Look at the tip of your nose and hold for up to twenty long breaths. Lower your legs to the floor during the final exhalation.

This important posture strengthens the arms and shoulders, and floods the brain with oxygenated blood.

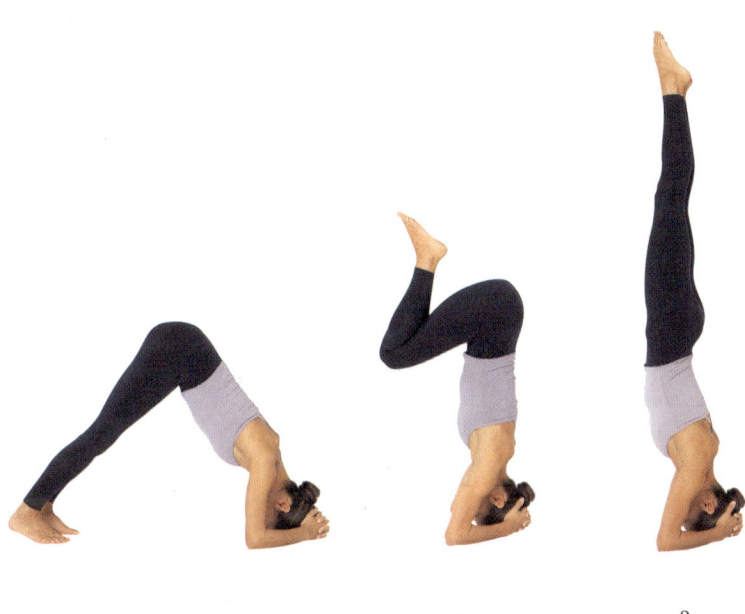

1   2   3

POSE OF THE CHILD
Balasana

Pose of the child is a counterpose to headstand and balances the effects of the inversions. It is also a classic yoga resting pose, which you can adopt at any point in your practice when you need a break. Based on the fetal position, pose o' the child is extremely calming and nurturing, and is useful if you are experiencing any difficult emotions – whether in your yoga practice or in your life generally. Begin by kneeling upright on the floor. Gently sit down on your heels, keeping your spine straight. Allow your arms to hang loosely at your sides and relax your hands. Exhaling, fold forward from your hips, bringing your chest to rest on your thighs and your head toward the floor, ahead of your knees. Let your hands slide backward toward your feet and your arms rest on the floor. Close your eyes and, keeping your breathing soft, even and relaxed, remain here for at least ten breaths (or half the time spent in headstand, if that is greater than ten breaths).

POSE OF THE CHILD

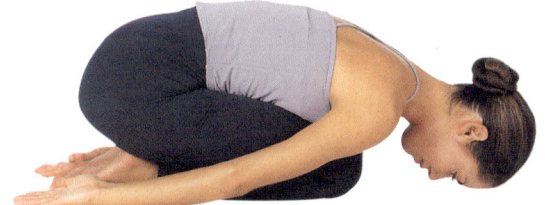

CROSS-LEGGED POSTURE
Padmasana (modified)

1 Begin in sitting ready pose. Inhaling, bring first one foot then the other in toward your groin, splaying your knees. Reach behind your back and cup your elbows with your hands. Exhaling, fold forward to the floor. Look to your "third eye" and hold for up to ten long breaths.

2 Inhaling, sit upright. Exhaling, place your hands just behind your hips, palms down with the fingers pointing forward. Inhaling, arch your back and lift your chest. Roll your head gently backward. Look toward your "third eye" and hold for up to ten long breaths.

3 Inhaling, sit upright. Exhaling, place your wrists on your knees, joining the thumbs and forefingers. Draw in your abdomen and lift through the crown of your head. Look at the tip of your nose and hold for up to ten long breaths. Exhaling, release the pose.

This meditative pose opens the hips, improves posture and circulation, and stills the mind and body to aid focus.

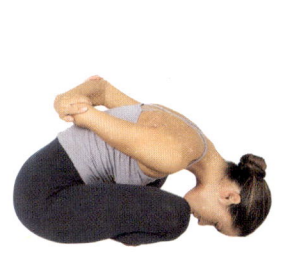

1

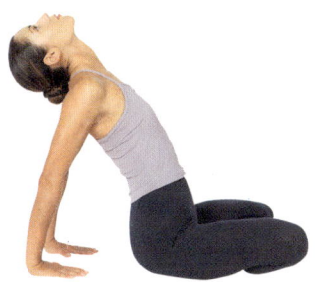

2

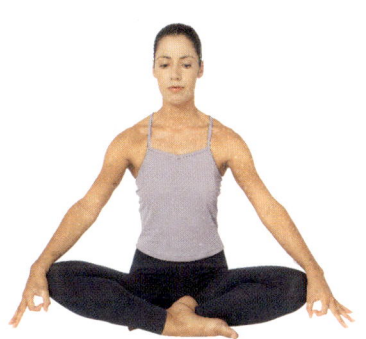

3

CORPSE POSTURE
Savasana

Always allow yourself time to perform this posture at the end of your practice. It will help to still your mind and realign your body, balancing the effects of the different postures in the sequences. Exhaling, lie down on your back with your arms by your sides, legs outstretched with the feet hip-width apart. Open your arms, turning your palms upward to help your chest open fully. Allow your feet to fall out to the sides. Make any adjustments necessary to ensure that your body is symmetrically aligned and you feel totally comfortable. Returning to normal breathing, close your eyes and relax, allowing the ground to support you as your body sinks into the floor. Focus on the different parts of your body in turn, beginning at your feet and moving toward your head. Work to dissolve any remaining tension. Finally, centre your mind within your body by bringing your attention to the relaxed rhythm of your breath. Remain in this position for at least five minutes.

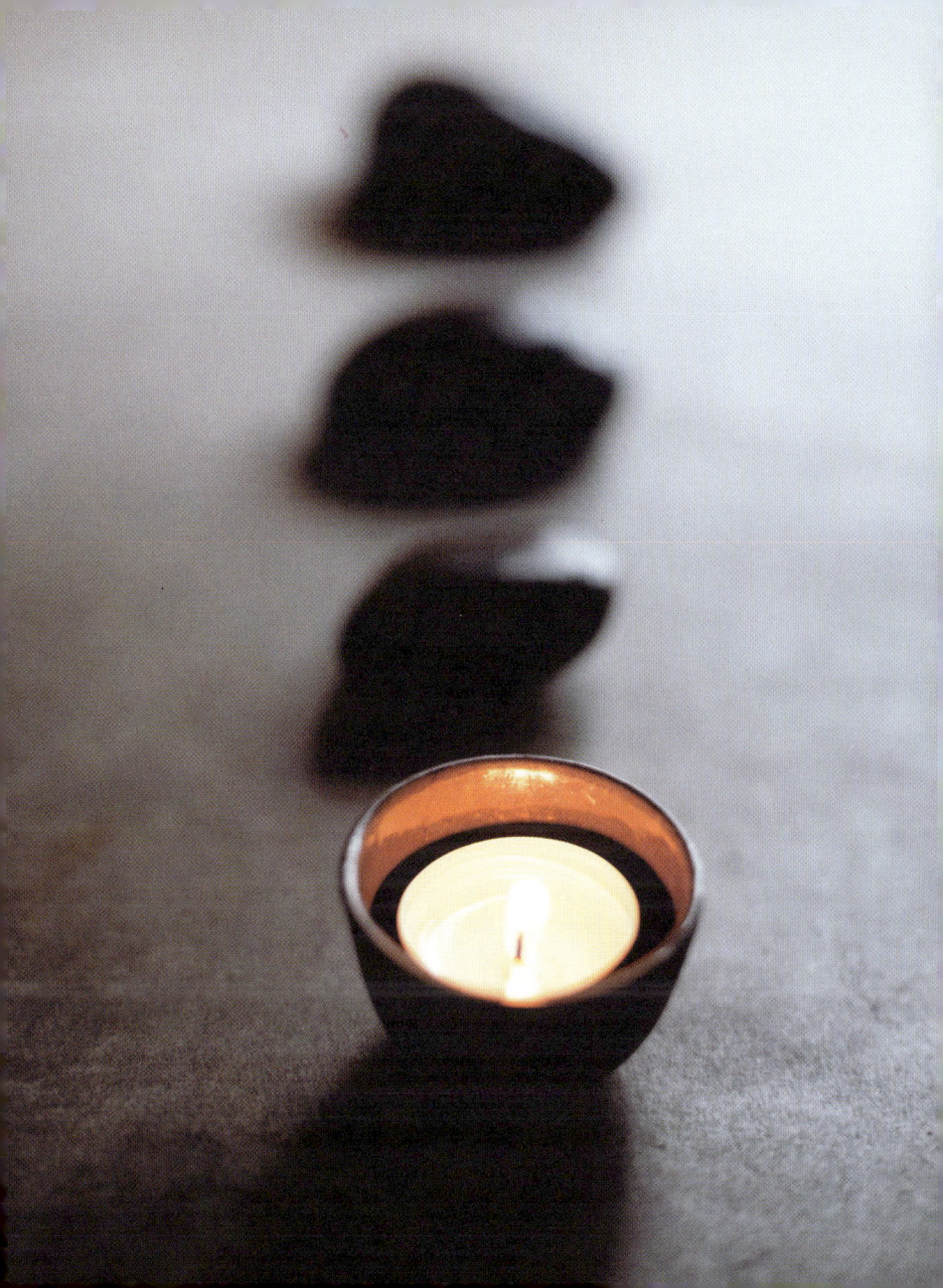

Above: the heavens – sky, sun, stars, moons, planets.
Below: the elements – space, air, fire, water, earth.
From these: the body – shape and form, vital breath,
digestive fire, blood and water, skeleton and flesh,
And the senses – hearing, touch, sight, taste, smell.
In contemplation of these sets of five,
The wise discovered that all things are holy.
One can complete the inner with the outer.

TAITTIRIYA UPANISHAD (7TH CENTURY BCE)

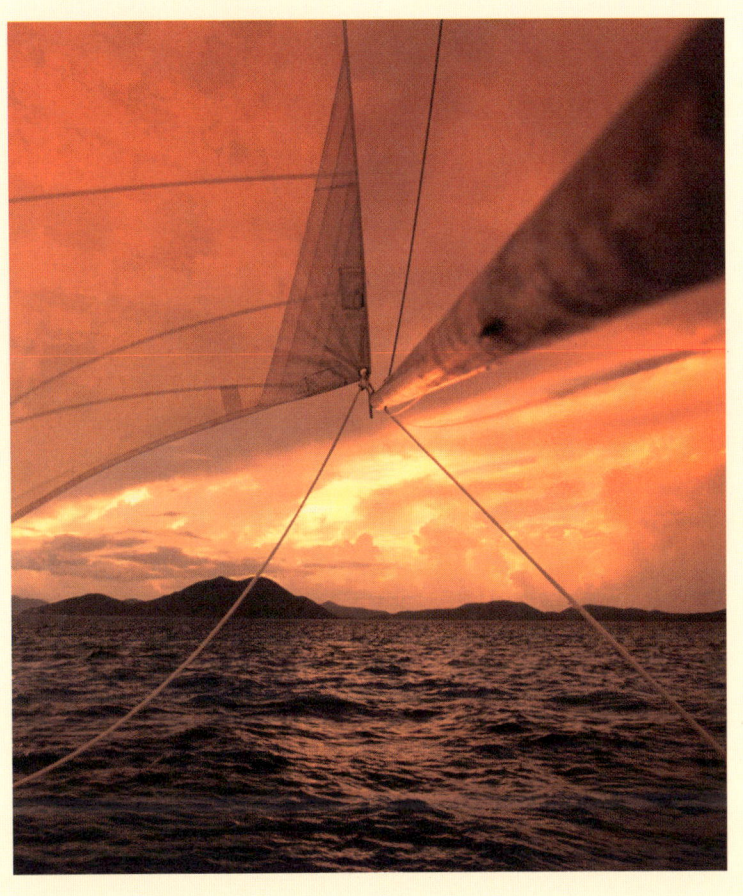

Chapter Six

ashtanga living

As we have seen, the initial aim of Ashtanga yoga (particularly of the Primary Series) is to cultivate a strong and supple body and a clear and focused mind through the practice of postures and controlled breathing techniques. It is often these elements that attract students to Ashtanga in the first place. However, achieving physical health is really only one aspect of yoga. Practising some of the other limbs outlined in Patanjali's *Yoga Sutras* (see p.12) is the key to introducing Ashtanga into all areas of our lives, both at home and at work.

Patanjali's eight limbs of yoga can be divided into two groups: the external limbs of *yama* (ethics), *niyama* (self-discipline), *asana* (posture practice) and *pranayama* (controlled breathing); and the internal limbs of *pratyahara* (withdrawal of the senses), *dharana* (concentration), *dhyana* (meditation) and *samadhi* (enlightenment or union with the true self).

In this chapter we begin with a discussion of the external limbs – the outward attitudes and practices that we should adopt toward ourselves, others and our surrounding environment. Once we have understood these, we can take our first steps on the more meditative path of yoga when we learn about the internal limbs, which take us on a journey of self-discovery and spiritual transformation.

THE EXTERNAL LIMBS

The external limbs of yoga involve physical effort and the conscious training of the mind and body in preparation for the internal limbs. In addition to *asana* and *pranayama* (discussed in previous chapters), the external limbs consist of *yama* and *niyama*, which are concerned with our personal, social and ethical attitudes and modes of behaviour.

Yama ethics

Yama is the first external limb and comprises five moral guidelines that teach us how to conduct our relationships with others and our environment. The first guideline is *ahimsa*, meaning nonviolence. This requires us to adopt an attitude of compassion toward all living things. Traditionally *ahimsa* involved the practice of vegetarianism, but today we can also understand it as a general attitude of respect to both ourselves and the world around us. Cultivate *ahimsa* in your yoga practice — remember to listen to your body with respect for your limitations; guard against the temptation to force your body into postures that are beyond its capabilities.

The second *yama* is the attitude of *satya* or truthfulness. Total honesty demands great courage but it is important to remember that telling a lie, however small, undermines our sense of worth – not only in the eyes of others, but more importantly in our own eyes, too.

Asteya (nonstealing) is the third *yama* and involves asking for no more than we need. For example, we should avoid taking anything, be it time, energy or wealth, from others unless it is freely given.

The fourth *yama* is *bramacharya*. Traditionally this was interpreted as the practice of chastity. Today we can understand it as a more general instruction to exercise moderation and self-restraint in all aspects of our lives.

Apariggraha is the fifth *yama* and means nonattachment or nonpossessiveness. A common pattern of human behaviour is to resist change by holding on to things, such as desires, people or material possessions, in an attempt to generate confidence and security. However, this state of being prevents us from living in a free and vital way. Instead it is better to welcome change, viewing it as an opportunity for growth and learning.

Niyama self-discipline

Niyama is the second external limb, comprising five principles that focus the mind on the inner quest for enlightenment. The first *niyama* is *sauca*, which means cleanliness or purity. *Sauca* refers not only to the cleanliness of our bodies, but also to our internal health. To practise *sauca* try to limit some of the toxins that you habitually ingest – not only alcohol and tobacco, but also the additives in processed foods, the pesticides sprayed on fruit crops, and the chemical residues in tap water.

The second *niyama* is *samtosa* (contentment). To achieve *samtosa* we need to focus our attention on the positive things that bless us in the present. This feeling of gratitude leads us to an automatic sense of abundance that we experience as contentment. Practising the meditation on p.118 will help you to experience this *niyama*.

The third *niyama* is *tapas*, which translates literally as "fire" or "heat". To live with an attitude of *tapas* is to demonstrate burning enthusiasm and commitment in all that we do – from mundane chores, such as cleaning the kitchen, to more challenging tasks, such as meeting deadlines. By channelling our energies in this way, we become more effective and feel happier as a result.

The fourth *niyama*, *swadhyaya*, means self-study. *Swadhyaya* involves developing awareness of our inner selves – of the unconscious urges that affect our behaviour and the beliefs that limit us – in order to expand our potential as human beings. To develop this *niyama* take time to reflect on your relationship with your yoga practice. What attitudes do you bring to each posture? You will probably find that they mirror your attitudes to life as a whole. This awareness is the first step to change.

The last of the *niyamas* is *ishwara-pranidhana*, which means devotion to a higher being or source of energy. If you are religious you can practise this *niyama* by worshipping the god of your chosen faith. Otherwise simply take some time to reflect in reverence and thanksgiving on the wonder of the world that surrounds you and the miracle that is your life.

CREATING CONTENTMENT

This visualization exercise will help you to develop *samtosa* (contentment) in your life. Practise it in the morning before rising – it will improve your mood for the rest of the day.

1 Sit or lie in a comfortable position on the floor with your back straight. Half-close your eyes and soften your gaze.
2 Consider the word contentment. What does it mean to you? How does it manifest itself within you – in your thoughts and feelings?
3 Think of a time in the past when you have experienced contentment. Perhaps while walking the dog, enjoying the warmth of sunshine in spring, or spending time with loved ones. Imagine yourself in that moment now, allowing the feelings of contentment to wash through you, filling your mind and permeating your body.
4 Allow your memories to drift away, but hold on to the sense of contentment that you have generated. When you feel ready, return your awareness to the present.

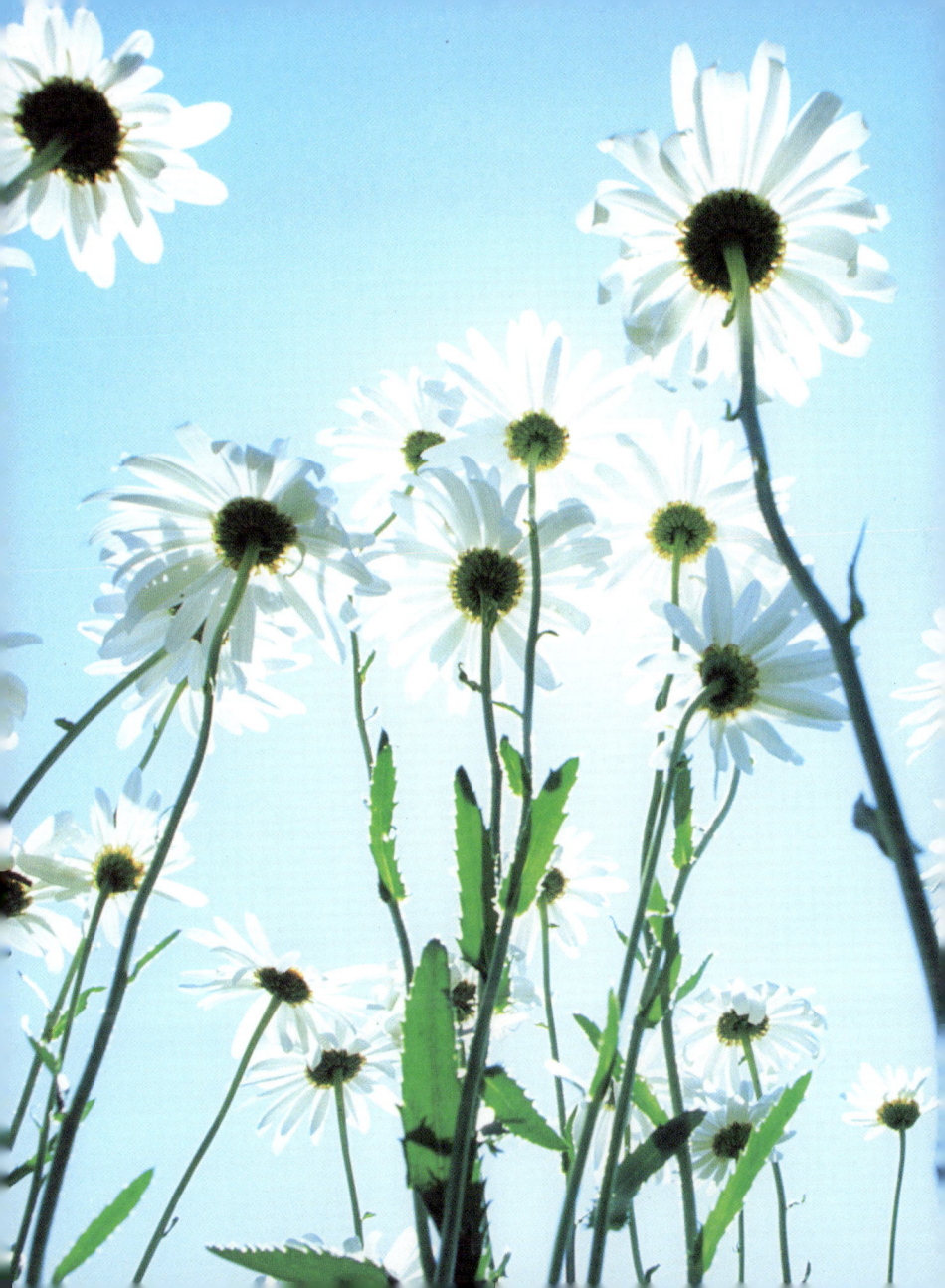

THE INTERNAL LIMBS

Once we have gained control over the mind and body by practising the external limbs of yoga, we are ready to develop yoga's internal limbs – *pratyahara*, *dharana*, *dhyana* and *samadhi*. These represent four stages of an inward journey toward spiritual enlightenment – the discovery of a point of stillness within the self and union with the universal consciousness.

Pratyahara withdrawal of the senses

Pratyahara is the first step on the road to meditation as we shift our attention from our external world, experienced through the senses, to our inner world. In Ashtanga yoga the *drishtis* (gaze points; see p.27) help us to develop this limb: by focusing on fixed points we limit what we can see around us.

Dharana concentration

When we are able to focus fully on the inner self, without becoming distracted by thoughts, emotions or the activities of others, we achieve the state of *dharana*. Practise the simple meditation on p.123 to help you to develop this limb.

Dhyana meditation

Dhyana describes a deep meditative state in which we lose the sense of separateness between being and doing. For example, when practising the *vinyasas* of Ashtanga yoga we reach *dhyana* when we become so absorbed in our practice that we experience self, movement and breath as one.

Samadhi union with the true self

Translated literally from the Sanskrit, *samadhi* means the "peace that passes all understanding". *Samadhi* is the highest meditative state – the point of "yoga" or "union" at which the yogi is said to have reached spiritual enlightenment. In this state any remaining sense of a separate self dissolves altogether as the yogi experiences oneness – a complete sense of connection to the universe and all that it contains.

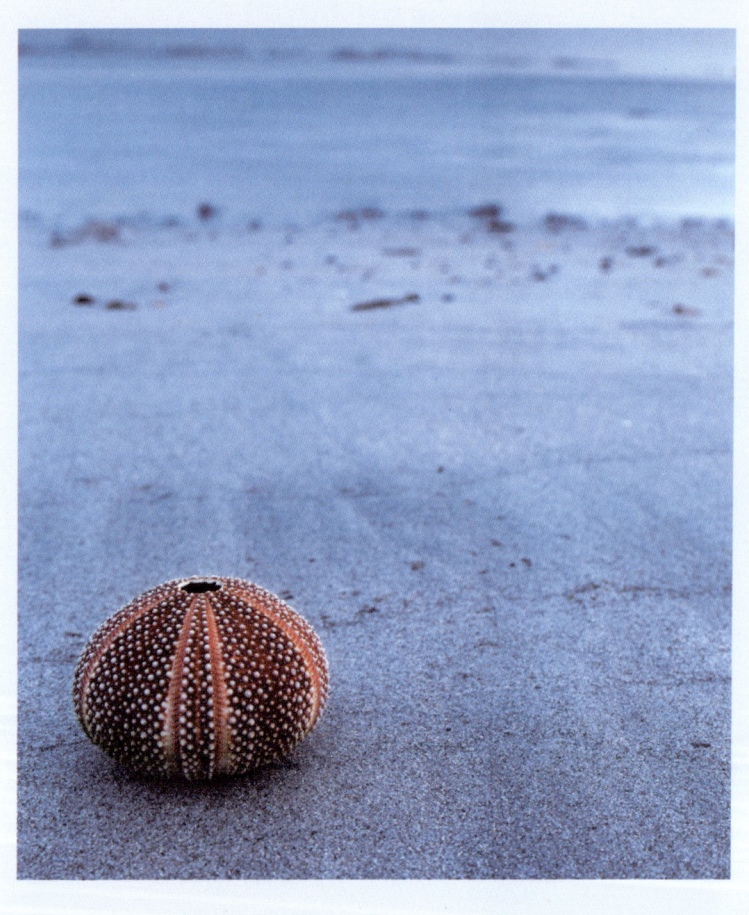

DEVELOPING DHARANA

Practise this simple meditation exercise at the end of your yoga session – it will help you to develop the concentration of *dharana*, freeing your mind from distractions and drawing your attention inward. Build up your meditation practice slowly. Start with ten minutes and increase the duration when you feel ready.

1 Sit in a comfortable position on the floor or on a chair, with your back straight and your eyes closed.

2 Focus each one of your senses on the physical action of breathing: listen to the rhythmic, rushing sounds of each inhalation and exhalation; feel the air on your skin as it passes in and out of your nostrils; experience the gentle expansion and contraction of your chest cavity; visualize each breath as it flows in and out of your lungs.

3 If you experience any distracting thoughts, do not feel frustrated. Simply observe each thought without judgment as it passes through your mind. Then return your attention to the breath once more.

When we live our lives with passion we crusade for our hearts: we dare to hope and to dream, without fearing failure; we are inspired with great purpose, our thoughts boundless and our minds open to embrace a world of limitless possibilities; hidden talents and abilities awaken in the face of challenge and excitement; and we discover ourselves to be greater people by far than we ever imagined we could be.

PATANJALI

YOGA SUTRAS (C.200BCE–C.200CE)

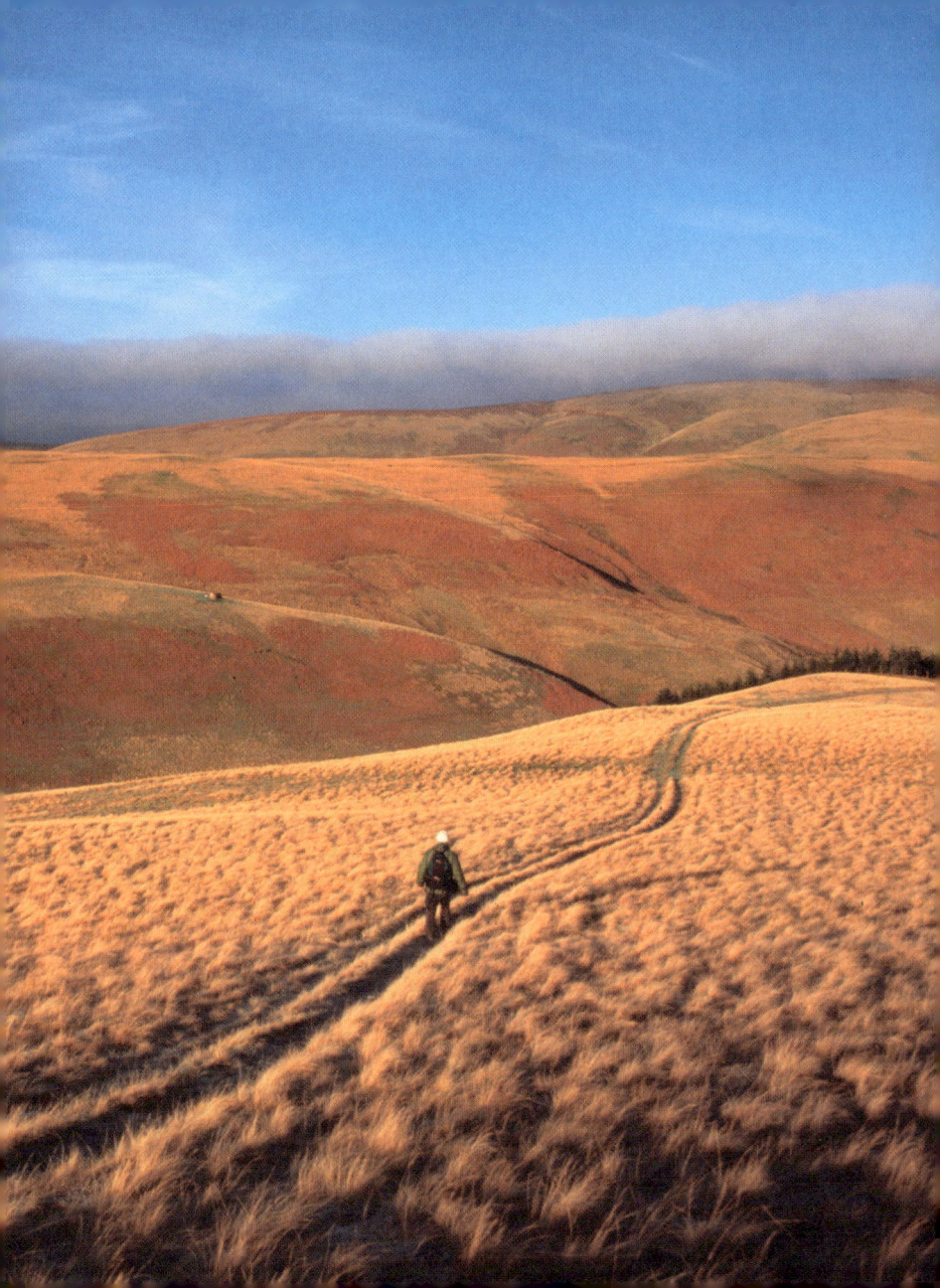

INDEX

PICTURE CREDITS AND ACKNOWLEDGMENTS

Picture Credits

The publisher would like to thank the following people, museums and photographic libraries for permission to reproduce their material. Every care has been taken to trace copyright holders. However, if we have omitted anyone we apologise and will, if informed, make corrections in any future edition.

Page 13 Makoto Saito/Photonica; **26** Mieko Kanasachi/Photonica; **33** Getty/Image Bank; **37** Yukari Ochiai/Photonica; **49** Steve Bloom Images; **73** Getty/Stone; **95** Getty/Stone; **109** Getty/Stone; **111** Getty/Image Bank; **119** Getty/Image Bank; **122** Getty/Image Bank; **125** Getty/Stone

Author's Acknowledgments

I dedicate this book to all of my teachers along my path so far, especially my first teachers: Francis, my mum; William, my dad; Michael and Sarah, my family. Kate – thank you for your heart, your kindness and your unwavering faith and support on the yoga path. Sarah and Nigel – thank you for the miles of smiles and just for being there. Lois – you taught me so much, how can I ever thank you enough? There are no words ... . Ross and the class of '88, we had the best of times. For precious moments and special lessons I thank in no particular order: Wendy, Ambro, Lino, Louly, Catherine, Nick and Helena, Barty, Angela, Russ and Caron, Noonie and Jiggster, to name but a few. For all my students, you continue to be my teachers and my inspiration. See you on the mat sometime.

Love and hugs, may peace and light be with you all, always.

OM Shanti Namaste

Anton ×

Publisher's Acknowledgements

Model: Kate Moore

Make-up artist: Tinks Reding